Sex in Your Marriage

Starved for Passion: Boosting Libido and Keeping Passionate Intimacy Alive in Committed Relationships

Ivan Rays

Table Of Contents

Introduction

Welcome to "Sex in Your Marriage," a thorough manual for improving closeness and contentment in your union. The purpose of this book is to give couples who want to foster a fulfilling relationship and enhance their sexual connection useful insights and techniques. Our goal is to enable you to confidently and clearly navigate the complexities of sexual intimacy by addressing common issues and providing helpful advice.

This book provides a road map to help you reach your objectives, whether you want to rekindle your passion, get past challenges, or just improve your relationship with your spouse. Come along with us as we set out on this journey together, learning fresh approaches to developing a more satisfying and active sexual relationship within your marriage.

My Story

As the writer of "Sex in Your Marriage," I offer a distinct viewpoint on the subject of sexual intimacy in partnerships. My interest in this field was sparked by my own personal experience navigating the challenges of my own marriage and trying to better understand and connect with my partner.

My spouse and I experienced difficulties in our sexual relationship, just like many other couples do. We experienced difficulties with intimacy, communication, and day-to-day stressors that frequently left us feeling empty and disengaged. I learned from this experience how crucial it is to have an honest conversation, to be vulnerable, and to make a conscious effort to cultivate a fulfilling and healthful sexual relationship.

I started my journey of self-discovery and education in the fields of sexology, relationship counseling, and personal development because I was passionate about assisting others in overcoming similar obstacles. To expand my knowledge of sexual intimacy and relational dynamics, I went to workshops, seminars, and sought advice from professionals in the field. I also immersed myself in research.

Equipped with fresh perspectives and understanding from my own experience, I embarked on a mission to educate people about "Sex in Your Marriage." I want to enable couples to overcome challenges, develop a stronger bond, and enjoy more fulfilling sexual relationships by using evidence-based concepts, doable tactics, and real-world examples.

By writing this book, I want to encourage couples to go out on their own paths of self-discovery and personal development, which will lead to a more vibrant, content, and profoundly fulfilling sexual relationship in their marriages.

Overview of the Book's Purpose and Structure
Purpose:
The goal of this book is to provide married couples the skills, information, and encouragement they need to successfully negotiate the challenges of sexual intimacy and forge a genuinely meaningful and rewarding bond. The goal of the book is to provide couples with the tools they need to overcome difficulties, communicate effectively, and rekindle love in their marriage by addressing common problems, misunderstandings, and roadblocks to sexual intimacy.

Structure:

The rational and approachable framework of the book leads readers on a voyage of discovery, comprehension, and personal development. Every chapter focuses on a different facet of sexual intimacy in marriage, providing advice, useful hints, and doable tactics to improve pleasure and connection. The following is how the chapters are arranged:

Introduction: Gives a synopsis of the goals and organization of the book and introduces the reader to the author's experience and viewpoint.

Understanding Sexual Intimacy in Marriage: Defines sexual intimacy, examines its significance in the context of marriage, and highlights typical difficulties that couples encounter.

Building a Foundation of Trust and Communication: Emphasizes the value of open communication and trust in developing a positive sexual connection throughout marriage.

Addressing Challenges in Sexual Intimacy: Provides advice on how to get beyond typical obstacles to sexual intimacy, such communication problems and traumatic experiences.

Cultivating Emotional and Physical Connection: Examines strategies for improving sexual closeness outside of the bedroom by strengthening emotional and physical ties.

Reigniting Passion and Rediscovering Desire: Offers doable advice and activities to help couples rekindle their romance and do new things together.

Embracing Change and Growth in Your Sexual Relationship: Encourages partners to welcome development and change in their sexual connection, understanding that change is an inevitable aspect of any committed relationship.

Overcoming Common Sexual Roadblocks: Discusses typical difficulties and barriers that couples may have in their sexual connection and provides advice and assistance for overcoming these hurdles.

Sustaining Long-Term Sexual Satisfaction: Outlines methods for maintaining long-term sexual contentment and happiness, emphasizing the need of self-care and milestone celebration.

Conclusion: Summarizes the main ideas and conclusions of the book, exhorts readers to put the knowledge to use, and ends with some parting advice on their path toward a sexual partnership.

Bonus: Includes worksheets or activities that couples may do together, a dictionary of important concepts pertaining to relationships and sexual intimacy.

With the help of this methodical approach, readers may work their way through the book and acquire insightful knowledge and useful skills to improve their sex life and fortify their marriage.

Chapter One

Understanding Sexual Intimacy in Marriage

We explore the complex terrain of sexual intimacy in your relationship in this chapter. Our objective is to shed light on the dynamics, obstacles, and transformative possibilities present in this intensely personal facet of partnership through perceptive investigation and useful advice. Come along as we help you understand the nuances of sexual intimacy so you can develop a deeper, more satisfying relationship with your partner.

Defining Sexual Intimacy

The closeness that partners in a love relationship have on a physical, emotional, and psychological level is referred to as sexual intimacy. It entails the sharing of intimate joys, weaknesses, and wants on both sides, resulting in a deep bond that transcends simple physical touch.

The qualities of sexual intimacy include trust, transparency, and a profound awareness of one another's needs and wants. It includes verbal displays of love, snuggling, kissing, and other intimate actions in addition to the act of sexual intercourse. A happy and healthy marriage must include sexual intimacy because it promotes emotional connection, relational happiness, and both spouses' general well-being.

The Real Meaning of Sexual Intimacy

There are several, intricate methods to characterize sexual intimacy in psychology. It's a notion that often surfaces in couple relationships, impacting not only the psychological and emotional but also the physical components.

Physical Connection: This includes all aspects of the actual sexual act, such as satisfaction, excitement, and touch. It's the interplay of bodies that offers closeness, enjoyment, and often a sense of unity.

Emotional Connection: The emotions of sexual intimacy are intimately associated with partner trust, empathy, and vulnerability. It creates a safe space where couples may express their desires, anxieties, and love without worrying about the consequences.

Psychological Intertwining: This section addresses expectations, sexuality-related attitudes, and perspectives that partners have on their sexual relationships. It highlights how the sex exchange relates to the partnership's overall structure and how it either reinforces or defies societal norms and personal aspirations.

Communication: For there to be a sexual connection, there must be an open discussion of one's sexual goals, wants, and limitations. This promotes understanding between the parties and a more fulfilling, consensual sexual relationship.

Mutual Growth and Exploration: Sexual intimacy usually involves a process of self-discovery and mutual improvement. It's a dynamic process that adapts to the two people's differing needs, viewpoints, and experiences as the relationship does.

Integration with Overall Intimacy: Sexual intimacy does not exist in a vacuum; it is a component of the partnership's overall closeness. Interacting with social, intellectual, and emotional links, adds to the general satisfaction and well-being of the couple.

Sexual intimacy is more than just physical actions; it is a deep and complicated phenomena in psychology. It's a dance of bodies, thoughts, and emotions that enhances the couple's overall connection and well-being while reflecting the larger dynamics of the relationship.

Importance of Connection and Fulfillment in Sexual Relationships

Beyond just physical gratification, sexual relationships need connection and fulfillment as essential components. They are about having a strong emotional and psychological bond with your mate.

Intimacy deepens a couple's relationship and increases trust when they feel connected to each other. It's important to feel appreciated, understood, and accepted by your partner in addition to the act itself. For both parties, this sensation of connectedness may heighten intimacy and make the encounter more satisfying.

Furthermore, a fulfilling sexual connection for both partners may be beneficial to the couple's general well-being. In order to sustain a solid and long-lasting relationship, it fosters sentiments of intimacy and fulfillment.

Essentially, a stronger feeling of intimacy, trust, and happiness between partners is facilitated by connection and fulfillment in sexual partnerships, which eventually enriches the relationship overall.

Nurturing Intimacy with Sexual Fulfillment

Matrimony is a deep connection between two people that goes beyond friendship, drawing them together in a journey of feelings, hopes, and experiences. The complexities of intimacy, which is the foundation of this union, is where physical, mental, and emotional ties come together to create a bond that can withstand life's adversities.

Among these components, sexual fulfillment is a crucial pillar, a potent force that not only amplifies the life of the relationship but also cultivates a more profound intimacy and connection that deepens with time.

The Nature of Intimacy:
Physical closeness alone is only one aspect of intimacy. It includes being emotionally open, communicating honestly, having similar goals, and accepting one's partner for who they are.

Within the framework of marriage, sexual fulfillment is a logical progression of this complex intimacy. It acts as a physical representation of the mental and emotional ties that bind two people together, serving as the embodiment of trust. In addition to enjoying a satisfying sexual experience, a couple that has a fulfilling sexual life is strengthening the fundamentals of their relationship.

Interaction and comprehension:
For a married couple to experience sexual fulfillment, there must be mutual understanding and open communication. An open discussion about one's needs, wants, boundaries, and even fears promotes a climate of acceptance and trust.

When partners are free to express their needs without fear of being judged, it creates an environment that encourages experimentation and discovery and enhances the overall sexual experience. Regular conversations about intimacy help to keep misunderstandings and resentment at bay, which in turn leads to a happier and healthier marriage.

Increasing the Emotional Connection:
Marriage-related sexual fulfillment fosters emotional closeness between partners. During physical intimacy, oxytocin, also known as the "love hormone," is released, which promotes feelings of attachment, closeness, and trust.

The emotional ties that couples develop via their shared experiences, difficulties, and personal development are enhanced by this physiological reaction. A satisfying sexual life provides a means for partners to show each other their love, care, and commitment to one another, strengthening their emotional bond and fostering a sense of security.

Adaptability in the Face of Difficulties:
Life's ups and downs, personal struggles, and external stressors can strain even the strongest relationships. These kinds of issues can arise in marriage. However, satisfying sex can serve as a barrier to keep these problems at bay.

Couples who prioritize their sexual fulfillment are better able to withstand the negative impacts of external stressors by accumulating a reserve of positive memories and emotions. The consoling warmth and support of each other's arms can provide a safe haven during trying times, reaffirming their commitment and serving as a reminder of their unique bond.

Probing and Venturing:
Couples go on a journey that is exclusive to their relationship as they explore their sexual desires together. This exploration journey is about letting go of inhibitions and accepting vulnerability in addition to finding what makes you happy.

A spirit of adventure and playfulness that is fostered by mutual exploration can revitalize a marriage by adding freshness and excitement to it. The desire to set out on this adventure together is indicative of a common dedication to personal development and fulfillment.

Keeping Away from Doldrums:
Like everything else in life, marriages need care and nurturing to be successful. Routines can develop over time, and the initial enthusiasm may wain.

The dynamic force of sexual fulfillment keeps a relationship from stagnating. A fulfilling sexual life provides excitement and passion that revitalize a marriage by reminding partners of the attraction and allure that first drew them to one another.

Managing Personal and Shared Needs:
Individual needs and preferences must be weighed against the needs of the partnership as a whole within the confines of a marriage. This also holds true for fulfilling sexual desires. It's critical for couples to find a balance between their own and their spouse's desires.

It takes empathy, compromise, and a thorough comprehension of one another's needs and boundaries to successfully navigate this negotiating process. The capacity to balance these elements creates a setting in which each partner feels heard and respected, strengthening the feeling of closeness and connection.

General Approach to Wellness:
The general well-being is enhanced by marital sexual fulfillment. Studies have connected regular sexual activity to several health benefits, including reduced stress, improved sleep, longer lifespans, and stronger immune systems.

Furthermore, enhanced mental health and a positive outlook are associated with the release of endorphins during sexual activity. Making their sexual relationship a priority enables partners to make investments in their general well-being, both individually and as a couple.

A vital link in the intricate fabric of marriage, sexual fulfillment establishes emotional, mental, and physical closeness. Its value goes beyond the pleasure of the senses to encompass exploration, trust, communication, and resilience.

A satisfying sex can rekindle the relationship, fortify emotional bonds, and provide a secure haven of intimacy during trying times. If a couple prioritizes sexual fulfillment, they can build a marriage that is based on understanding, connection, and a shared growth journey.

Common Challenges Faced by Couples in Maintaining Sexual Intimacy

Problems that could be keeping you and your partner from having as much sex as you could. There is a widespread misconception that men are consistently more interested in sex than women. However, there are a lot of things that can actually prevent a man from wanting sex, and if his wife doesn't know about these things, it can be hurtful and confusing. Here are just a handful to think about:

Medications: According to therapists, this is the most common and often ignored cause of decreased male libido. Drugs, both prescription and over-the-counter, have the power to suppress a man's desire for sex. If you think this is one of the causes, talk to your doctor about potential remedies.

Depression: Even though depression is the most common psychological problem in the world, this is the second most often ignored issue in men. It truly kills sexual desire. Once more, if you suspect that you may be depressed, see your doctor.

Watching Porn: An increasing number of honorable men and women are suffering because of porn. If this is a problem for you, own up to it and get support. By holding yourself accountable and seeking professional counseling support when needed, you can combat this threat and bring back the closeness in your marriage.

Male sexual dysfunction can also be caused by drugs or alcohol, erectile dysfunction, illness, aging, or pain, relationship issues or unresolved conflict in your marriage, childhood experiences or abuse, sexual inexperience or performance anxiety, and plain old stress. However, there are always things you can do to lessen the impact of these problems. Instead of enduring the pain in silence and allowing your sexual life to stagnate, assess yourself to find out what could be the source of the issue.

Frequently cause of sexual problems in women.:

Among them are:

Psychological: These may result from feelings of inferiority complex, marital conflict, anxiety, guilt, depression, or fear. Past sexual trauma may also have a connection to them. Did you grow up witnessing sexual abuse? Have you ever experienced sexual assault? Before you were married, were you and your spouse promiscuous? Have any of you ever engaged in pornographic activities? If you said "yes" to any of these inquiries, it's probable that your sexual reactivity is being impacted by prior experiences.

Physiological: Some women experience pain during sexual activity because there is not enough lubrication, not enough stimulation, an infection, or another physical reason. Additionally, some medications and chronic illnesses can significantly reduce one's desire for sex. Hormonal abnormalities, vitamin shortages, hypothyroidism, menopause, tiredness, and childbirth are a few more physical factors that may exist. Make sure you talk to your doctor about any concerns you have if you believe your issue may have a medical origin.

Relationship-based: It's a fact that a husband's attitudes and behavior have a significant impact on his wife's sexual experience; I don't mean to put men in a bad light here. When a woman feels safe, comfortable, respected, loved, and valued, she reacts to her husband's advances more readily and naturally. However, she will almost certainly lose her sexual ardor if she feels like she's just being used.

How do you and your spouse interact outside of the bedroom?

Does he prioritize your needs and worries over his own?

Does he give you compliments, try to improve your perception of yourself, and offer to help in any way that he can?

It could be time for a heart-to-heart conversation without placing blame or shame.

These lists, which apply to both men and women, are by no means all-inclusive. For numerous couples, being overly busy is the biggest obstacle to having a more satisfying sexual life. Regain control of your marriage if that is the case. If you really must, schedule some sex! Although scheduling sex in your calendar may not seem romantic, it might be necessary if you're going through a particularly busy time in your life.

Other typical examples of challenges are as follows:
Communication Issues: Miscommunications and dissatisfaction may arise when inclinations, fears, and wishes for sexual intimacy are not communicated in a clear and unambiguous way.

Mismatched Libidos: Differing levels of sexual frequency and desire may cause one or both partners to feel unworthy or unacceptcd, which may cause stress and unpleasant relationships.

Stress and Fatigue: Setting sex as a priority may be challenging since stressors like hectic schedules and hard work can lower libido and energy levels.

Routine and Monotony: A person's enjoyment of sex may be diminished if they get used to patterns or rituals, which may cause boredom and a lack of enthusiasm in the bedroom.

Body Image Issues: A person's confidence and self-esteem may suffer as a result of insecurities about their physical appearance or body image, which may make them uncomfortable or unable to engage in sexual activity.

Past Trauma or Emotional Baggage: Intimacy and trust might be hampered by unresolved emotional difficulties or past trauma, which can limit one's capacity to fully participate in sexual activities.

Lack of Time and Prioritization: Couples with hectic schedules and conflicting goals might find it difficult to spend quality time together, which could limit their chances of intimacy and connection.

External Stressors: External variables that impact sexual intimacy include significant life changes, parenting duties, and financial hardship. These elements might perhaps increase the stress level of the relationship.

To tackle these obstacles, a couple must be willing to collaborate, have empathy, and be open to open communication. A therapist or counselor may be a valuable resource for negotiating these challenges and enhancing sexual connection in a relationship.

Chapter Two

Building a Foundation of Trust and Communication

Let's shed light on the two most important components of a successful marriage in this chapter: communication and trust. We explore the crucial role they play in creating intimacy and provide useful tips and techniques to reinforce this basis. Let's through the nuances of developing open communication and trust, enabling you and your spouse to deepen your connection and fortify your bond.

Establishing Trust and Open Communication

A crucial aspect of intimacy and sexual activity is communication with a partner. Increased sexual comfort and enjoyment may result from being honest and open with one another. Many find it challenging to have successful conversations about sex with their spouses. When someone attempts to talk about their wishes but isn't sure how to articulate them, it might cause some pain. The following points provide information about methods of sexual communication.

Be Clear:

It may be difficult, but there are many reasons why it's important to have an exact and lucid discussion with a partner before having sex. Communication is an ongoing process in which people learn about and respect each other's needs, preferences, boundaries, and desires. More pleasant conversations during intercourse may be facilitated by clear communication prior to intercourse.

An unambiguous consent process is the foundation of effective sexual communication. Even while it's essential, answering "yes" or "no" is just one step in the process of having open discussion about sexual activity. It all boils down to helping each other completely comprehend the needs, desires, and wants of the other. Examples of communication include talking about whether or not foreplay is necessary for sexual activity and whether or not sex toys are wanted and, if so, which ones. You may also decide to talk about your sexual wants if that is how you both feel comfortable doing so.

Vocal communication is not usually required for sexual communication. Body language, which is conveyed via the use of one's hands, eyes, lips, body, and facial expression, is another essential aspect of communication. Phrases like "touch here," "touch there," "harder," "softer," "more," "less," "faster," and "slower" may all be used to communicate your sexual desires. Though they may all be used to communicate concepts succinctly and effectively, these phrases can also cause confusion.

For instance, "faster" might be interpreted as meaning "harder." This is the point when effective communication becomes essential to having a fulfilling sexual experience with your partner. It's critical to communicate when sexual activities need to be changed or enhanced and to appreciate when they are going well. Useful expressions include "right there," "that feels good," and "keep doing that."

Nonverbal communication is another means of communicating during sexual activity, as was previously mentioned. For example, you may place your hand exactly where your partner wants it, push your body against theirs, or vary the pace, force, and tone of your touch and movement. Pleasure and desire may rise when communication is facilitated by both verbal and nonverbal clues.

Be Positive:
The golden rule is applicable not just in the bedroom but also in larger society. In other words, "the streets and the sheets are equally subject to the golden rule."1. These proverbs emphasize the value of kindness, patience, support, compassion, and helpfulness while educating partners about sexuality. Being patient and cheerful while avoiding dwelling too much on criticism or annoyance is an essential component of successful sexual communication.

Many people find it very unpleasant to discuss sexual activity, but as was already said, communication is essential to ensuring that both parties have the knowledge necessary to participate in consenting sexual activity. This part of the Golden Rule is particularly crucial when it comes to making required adjustments for disabilities. It is crucial to continue being kind, encouraging, and patient, in part because sex isn't always automatic and may take some additional time to arrange and identify the "key spots" that might trigger an orgasm.

In order to have open and honest conversation with your spouse during a time when both of you may feel vulnerable, try to be more positive than negative when you speak. Talk to them and explain why you did not like something, and instead of concentrating too much on something you may not have loved, be helpful and constructive.

A woman with a handicap could discover, for example, that the pressure was too strong or too light, that a certain position hurt, or that there was no pleasure. Kind, nonjudgmental communication on such matters demonstrates your understanding of the other person's perspective. It is imperative that individuals respect boundaries and take into account their partner's needs and desires.

Listen and Ask Questions:
As humans, we typically start formulating our own answers while others are still speaking, making it difficult to actually "listen" to them. To truly listen to your partner, you need to focus entirely on what they are saying and offer your undivided attention.

Sayings such as "I need you to press harder on my nipples when you are using your fingers during foreplay, to make me happy" are probably attempts at self-prediction if you hear your partner say them. Another way to gain a deeper understanding of your partner's perspective is to ask follow-up questions.

How to Address Differences:
Most people discover that their expectations don't always match reality when they start a relationship. It is important to address this subject in an open and sensitive manner. It is believed that open communication about one's sexual preferences improves feelings of intimacy and increases sexual satisfaction.

To properly communicate their desires to their partner, each person should take the time to consider what it is that they truly want. A kind and compassionate approach to bonding is to gradually ease into compromise. Trying out new sexual approaches can demonstrate to your partner that you are willing to develop a more intimate relationship. This could take the form of one person disclosing their sexual preference one week, followed by a weekly rotation to try something new. This quantity doesn't have to be a set amount; it can vary for every couple based on how often they engage in sexual activity.

When to Seek Professional Help:
Sex therapy or couples and marriage counseling can be helpful if you're finding it difficult to talk openly with your partner about sex. When talking about sex negatively impacts the dynamic of the relationship or when it frequently sparks an argument, seeking professional assistance may be necessary.

Couples who wish to feel more at ease in their own space can benefit greatly from online therapy options. An online therapist directory can help couples who might not live together find telehealth appointments that work with their schedules and living arrangements.

Indications that counseling is needed:
Indications that counseling might improve the intimacy in your relationship include:

- [ ] When having sexual conversations negatively affects the relationship

- [ ] An overall absence of closeness

- [ ] Inadequate physical or emotional bonding

☐ Communication difficulties

☐ Disagreement regarding intimacy and sex

☐ Adultery

☐ Insufficient trust

Although discussing sex with your partner can cause anxiety, it's necessary to keep lines of communication open and your relationship strong. Everyone should concentrate on having honest communication with their partner and have reasonable expectations. Instead of comparing themselves to friends or people they see on social media or television, couples should just concentrate on what works for them. All that matters is that they are content with their sexual relationship.

Discussing Sexual Needs and Desires

Speaking about needs and desires is one of the most crucial steps towards developing a happy and healthy sexual relationship within a marriage. However, it can also be a sensitive and sometimes challenging topic for couples to talk about.

How to Discuss Sex with Your Significant Other: It can improve your relationship when you bring up the subject of sex with your spouse when they are both feeling open and at ease. Developing a strategy and focusing on one problem at a time will help to move the conversation along, as will making your partner feel comfortable with your openness and empathy.

Why It's Important to Talk About Sex With Your Partner:
Sex strengthens the bond between partners and builds a closer connection in romantic or sexual relationships. Each partner can learn how to meet the needs of the other and return love and intimacy by having candid and open discussions about sex.

By creating a more stable and secure dynamic where people feel safe and can trust each other more, talking about sex can increase both the physical and emotional intimacy between partners. More intimate sex and higher levels of sexual satisfaction result from increased feelings of intimacy brought about by sexual communication.

Topics to Discuss When Talking About Sex:
To strengthen their bond and foster trust, partners should talk about things that are important to them when having sex. Recall that no topic is right or wrong. The talk should go easily as long as you concentrate on listening and are honest.

Topics to cover when discussing sex:
When talking about sex with your partner, you should talk about the following topics;

Modifications to Libido: Anybody can experience changes in libido at any time. It's crucial to talk to your partner about libido fluctuations in order to explain newly conflicting sex drives or explain why you might not be feeling as in the mood. A person's libido may be impacted by certain medical conditions, insecurities, stress, and sexual disorders, which can result in a dead bedroom, that's, lack of sexual activity. If you don't communicate these changes, they may have a long-term impact on your relationship as a whole.

Crying During Intercourse: While crying during sex or after an orgasm is perfectly normal for some people, you should take some time to talk about how you're feeling with your partner.

Desiring to Give Something New a Shot: Finding new tastes and preferences in sex can be a thrilling experience. Telling your partner that you want to try something different can help avoid problems from boring sex, so don't be scared to do so. If you concentrate on what you like and why this would turn you on, it will be easier to discuss new sexual ideas or fantasies you might want to try.

Lack of Intimacy: It is essential to your relationship's success that you talk about the lack of sexual intimacy in it. You can have a more open discussion about any changes that need to be made to increase your level of satisfaction when you address the degree of intimacy you require to feel loved, engaged, and sexual. Ignoring a lack of closeness in your relationship can make you feel more and more apart from each other, which can lead to more serious problems.

Practicing Safe Sex: Before getting intimate, every couple should talk about safe sex practices. Prior to your sexual relationship developing, you should take steps to protect both yourself and your partner. Talk about how you plan to have safe sexual relations so that you can both establish sensible limits. You can always start the conversation with a question if you're uncomfortable doing so. By posing questions to your partner, you demonstrate your interest in both resolving your worries and finding out about their needs.

Sexual Fantasies: Sexual fantasies can be a difficult subject to discuss. Sharing your fantasies can make you feel exposed because you are sharing your private thoughts. But fantasies about sex are quite normal. As long as one's fantasies do not endanger others, there should be no shame associated with having them. You might begin to feel more comfortable and secure in the relationship as you both become more vulnerable and reveal your deepest desires. When two people explore intimacy together, these talks can strengthen trust and their relationship.

If your partner expresses a sexual fantasy, you are under no obligation to acquiesce if it makes you uncomfortable. But, you can strengthen your bond both inside and outside of the bedroom by confiding in your partner about your deepest feelings without fear of rejection or condemnation.

When Sex Isn't Appropriate: Having a conversation about when sex is inappropriate aids in setting up sound boundaries. When it comes to when they want or don't want to have sex, everyone may feel differently. Some partners believe that having sex is inappropriate after an argument, when someone is ill or has mental health concerns, or when they are feeling less connected. Maintaining communication with your partner about your expectations regarding what constitutes appropriate and inappropriate sex is crucial.

Family Planning: Family planning will eventually come up as a topic that should be discussed when you are in a relationship. It is okay for each partner to express when or if they hope to begin family planning. If you and your spouse have different expectations, this should be discussed in an honest and open dialogue. You can talk about sex and how you want to meet those planning needs, depending on when you both feel ready to begin family planning.

When to Talk to Your Partner About Sexual Issues:
It is best to discuss sex with your partner in a setting where you both feel comfortable and supported. It's not a good idea to discuss sex with your partner during a fight because this can lead to long-term issues and insecurities.

It is advisable to have a conversation about sex before you even begin to explore each other sexually. Talking about touchy or awkward topics more frequently will make you feel closer and make it simpler to work out any problems that may come up in your relationship.

The right time to talk about sex is:

When both of you are at ease: Select a moment when you are both feeling relaxed and joyful. This will be the ideal opportunity to talk honestly about a delicate subject.

When you experience a physical and emotional connection: Select a moment when you both experience a sense of physical and emotional connection. By talking about your vulnerabilities, this will help you feel less intimidated.

When you're ready to speak: Don't hesitate to speak up about significant subjects like sex. Make plans to discuss your sexual desires and worries with your spouse.

Prior to talking about sex with your spouse, you ought to:
Do not do these;

Don't talk about sexual issues after having sex: Talking about sexual issues after sex can come across as judgmental. The emotional impact of these discussions can be lessened by bringing up sex when you are both spending quality time together and when you feel comfortable talking about it. You run the risk of making yourself or your partner feel more insecure and vulnerable if you wait until after sexual activity.

Never surprise your partner: At the outset of intimacy, you want to be honest with your partner to avoid taking them by surprise. Talk to your partner in a calm and collected manner about the things you enjoy and find offensive. They might feel insecure and deceived if you wait months afterward and think you have withheld information from them. Some couples' trust may be broken by this.

Select a neutral venue for the conversation: To keep the conversation as calm as possible, it's crucial to pick a neutral space to talk about any personal or delicate subject. It's important to choose a place that both of you feel comfortable. To enable you to concentrate on what your partner is sharing with you, this location should ideally not be overly busy or noisy.

In order to ensure that neither of you feels as though your privacy is being violated, you want to be aware of how many people are around you. Intimate spaces in your home, like your bedroom, are typically where you spend time together. Engaging in a conversation such as this one in your bedroom could upset the balance of the space and cause your partner to feel uncomfortable.

Ways to Have a Sexual Discussion with Your Spouse:
Here are pointers for talking to your partner about sex:

Pick a Time: Setting up a conversation time helps both partners prepare their thoughts and work through their emotions. Look for days or times when you know you'll be more at ease and relaxed when making your schedule. It is advisable to avoid trying to have a conversation about anything during the busiest times of the day, such as right after work. Rather, schedule some time to talk about your emotions when you're both at ease and not in a rush.

Be Sensitive to Their Feelings: It's crucial to consider other people's feelings since talking about any intimate subject can make people feel more exposed. Use words or phrases that reassure your partner when you share your thoughts. You can begin with the things you already like and gradually work your way up to the changes you would like to see. To make sure your partner feels heard and understood, you can use reflective listening and validation to improve your relationship communication skills.

Ask questions: It's always beneficial to ask questions because it allows your partner to elaborate. When you ask questions, you stop making assumptions and receive truthful answers, you are free to fill in the blanks with your own negative story or anxious thoughts. You can have better sex if you ask your partner about intimacy and what they would like. It demonstrates your willingness to listen and consider novel concepts that you are posing these questions.

Begin with caution: It's crucial to start a delicate conversation slowly and introduce the topic gradually. You can set up the ideal environment for discussing intimacy by arranging the furniture and creating a serene, quiet area. It is not necessary to create a sexually charged environment in order to minimize strong emotions; rather, you just need to create a calm environment.

Express Your Emotions: It's recommended to share and build relationships because this is a delicate subject that could make people feel exposed. You can establish rapport and get your partner to open up by talking to them about how you feel. To facilitate a more natural flow of the conversation, begin by sharing your feelings. It's usually a good idea to put your feelings in writing before discussing them with your partner.

Don't be judgemental: Your partner may withdraw and lose trust in you if you make judgments. You can reassure your partner that they are in a safe place by refusing to pass judgment. When you discuss sex with your partner, try not to criticize them because it will come across as judgmental. Commencing your speech with affirmations and praises will assist you in staying on target and communicating from an open and thankful place.

Have Patience: Because it's a delicate and vulnerable subject, having patience with your partner is essential. Your partner will feel more comfortable expressing themselves if you create a safe space where you are willing to listen and do not put pressure on them to share. Another thing you can do is try to put yourself in their position. Silence the critical voice inside of you and give yourself permission to hear without responding.

Employ personalized sentences: You can concentrate on your needs rather than what your partner isn't providing for you by using "I" statements. This lessens the likelihood of experiencing defensiveness. This lets you accept responsibility for your actions and lessens the blame you might otherwise place on your spouse. It's easier to express what you want when you use "I" statements.

Remain Focused and Explicit: It's critical to maintain emotional awareness in order to avoid sending contradictory messages and misunderstandings. You can stay on topic and remember what you want to say if you prepare for the talk. Instead of circling back and forth because you're not sure what you need, try your hardest to be explicit about it. You can communicate in a clear and concise way by practicing being forceful with your language.

Have a kind and open mind when you approach the conversation: Your partner will feel that you are acknowledging their needs and feelings if you are kind and open with them. Empathy maintains an emotional connection between you and your partner. Remaining receptive enables you to pause and avoid responding negatively at first. You can show your partner empathy and understanding by keeping an open mind. This demonstrates to them your willingness to hear what they have to say and to listen to them.

Establishing a Supportive and Safe Space for Sexual Exploration

It is imperative to create a secure and encouraging atmosphere for sexual exploration prior to a couple feeling confident enough to talk about their choices and desires:

Encourage clarity and truthfulness: Build a relationship where both parties feel free to freely express their needs and desires in order to avoid suspicion or criticism. One aspect of this is encouraging empathy, understanding, and respect between people.

Unambiguous Communication: Promote open and sincere dialogue about boundaries, desires, and sexual orientation. As you respectfully and openly voice your own desires, be prepared to actively listen to your partner's needs and preferences.

Accommodate Each Other's Boundaries: When it comes to sexual exploration, it's critical to honor each other's comfort zones and boundaries. Be open to your partner's boundaries and transparent about what you are comfortable with.

Accept your vulnerable nature: Emotional transparency and vulnerability are common components of sexual exploration. Establish a secure environment where both partners can express their most private fantasies and desires without worrying about being rejected.

Exercise Objectivity: When talking about your sexual preferences and desires, try not to be critical or judgmental. Rather, approach the discussion with acceptance, curiosity, and a desire to jointly explore novel avenues.

Make Consent a Priority: Any sexual interaction requires consent. Consent should be freely given and withdrawn by both partners without coercion. Honor each other's choices and put mutual satisfaction and consent first at all times.

Playfulness and Experimentation: Take a playful and inquisitive approach to sexual exploration. Examine novel pursuits, methods, or imaginations in a spirit of adventure and with an open mind.

Establish a Calm Environment: Make your space comfortable and relaxing to create the ideal atmosphere for sexual exploration. To improve the atmosphere, try turning down the lights, turning on calming music, or lighting scented candles.

Respect every person's wishes: Even if someone's goals and choices differ from your own, respect and support each other's choices. Recognize that every person is unique and that you should cherish the range of experiences that each person brings to the relationship.

When help is needed, ask for it: Couples who experience difficulties creating a safe and supportive space for sexual exploration should not put off getting assistance from a therapist or counselor who specializes in sexual health and intimacy. To enhance sexual exploration and satisfaction in a partnership, a qualified expert can provide guidance, aid in communication, and offer resources and strategies.

Couples can create a secure and encouraging environment for sexual exploration that promotes intimacy, connection, and mutual satisfaction in their relationship by placing a high priority on trust, communication, respect, and consent.

Chapter Three

Addressing Challenges in Sexual Intimacy

Let's address the obstacles that can occur in a married couple's sexual intimacy in this chapter. From mismatched libidos to communication problems, we break down typical problems and provide workable answers. Join us as we explore these challenges, offering solutions and advice to get past them and promote a more satisfying and peaceful sexual relationship.

Overcoming Communication Barriers in the Bedroom

Not everyone feels at ease discussing sex with their significant other. For a better sex life, we teach you how to communicate more effectively during sex.

Sexual activity is not the only aspect of sex. It also includes a small amount of flirting, some foreplay, and conversation about sex and pleasure. Not only can effective sexual communication increase the enjoyment of your sex life, but it can also promote intimacy, establish mutual satisfaction, and build trust. However, few people enjoy discussing sex. They don't feel at ease or they are shy. The secret is to make an effort to communicate with your partner more sexually.

What is sexual communication?

The sharing of verbal and nonverbal cues between partners about their sexual experiences, boundaries, desires, and preferences is referred to as sexual communication. It requires the capacity to listen intently and sympathetically to a partner's needs and worries, as well as the ability to express one's boundaries and desires in a clear and concise manner.

Couples who express dissatisfaction with their sexual life are likely to blame one another for poor communication and poor sexual expression. Therefore, having sexual communication in a relationship is crucial. It is essential for developing intimacy as well as elevating relationship satisfaction in general. People establish a safe space for honesty and vulnerability by being upfront about their preferences, boundaries, and desires. This deepens the emotional connection between them. According to the expert, couples who communicate openly and honestly about their sexual needs are better able to handle consent concerns, negotiate sexual activities, and develop a fulfilling and satisfying sexual connection.

Why is sexual communication difficult for some couples?

Some people might find it effortless to discuss sex, while others might find it challenging. These are a few of the reasons:

I.   Individuals may be reluctant to bring up their sexual needs with their partner because they are ashamed or embarrassed about talking about them for fear of being rejected or judged.

II. Barriers to open communication about sexual desires and preferences can arise from societal taboos and cultural norms surrounding sex.

III. An individual's comfort level with sexual communication can be greatly impacted by past experiences, such as traumatic or unpleasant sexual encounters.

IV.   Difficulties in communicating sexually can be attributed to variations in assertiveness and communication styles between partners.

V.   Insecurities, trust issues, and unresolved relationship conflicts are examples of underlying issues that can make it more difficult to communicate sexually.

What are the ways to improve sexual communication with a partner?

Since it's crucial, here are some pointers to improve your sexual communication with your partner:

Establish an environment of emotional stability and trust: Create a safe, judgment-free environment where both partners feel free to communicate their desires, thoughts, and anxieties without fear of rejection or retaliation.

Start a candid discussion: Start having discussions about sexuality outside of the bedroom to ease tensions and provide space for inquiry. Talk calmly and respectfully about things like boundaries, fantasies, sexual preferences, and concerns.

Engage in attentive listening: Without interrupting or making snap judgments, pay close attention to your partner's thoughts, feelings, and desires. In order to create empathy and understanding in your relationship, give them credit for their feelings and experiences.

Appropriate statement selection: Express your own needs, wants, and feelings through "I" statements rather than assigning blame or drawing conclusions about your relationship.

Be clear and concise: To prevent miscommunication or misunderstandings, express your sexual preferences, boundaries, and expectations in clear terms. According to the expert, you can help your partner better understand your desires by giving specific examples or suggestions.

Request feedback: Ask your spouse for their thoughts on their own experiences and aspirations. It will guarantee that you both feel satisfied and appreciated in the sexual relationship.

Look for nonverbal clues: During sexual encounters, pay attention to non-verbal cues such as body language, gestures, and facial expressions to gain a better understanding of your partner's desires and reactions. Be sensitive to their cues in order to foster a greater sense of enjoyment and connection between you both.

Respect limits and consent: Give your partner's consent and agreement top priority before engaging in any intimate acts, and honor their limits and preferences when it comes to sexual activity. Establish clear boundaries and be open and honest about consent in order to ensure that both partners have a safe and pleasurable sexual experience.

Be understanding and patient with others: If your partner finds it difficult to discuss their sexuality or has a history of trauma or insecurities, be patient and understanding with them. Talk to them with compassion and understanding, and refrain from pressuring them to reveal more information than they are comfortable with.

Seek professional help when required: You might want to see a therapist or counselor who specializes in relationship and sexual health issues if your problems with sexual communication don't get better after trying a few different approaches. To improve sexual satisfaction and communication in a partnership, a qualified specialist can provide guidance, support, and tools.

Consistently practice: As with any skill, sexual communication gets better with use. Try to have regular discussions with your partner about sexuality, and be willing to grow and learn from each other as you work through the challenges of your relationship.

You can develop a deeper understanding, connection, and fulfillment in the sexual relationship by putting these strategies into practice; this will increase intimacy and satisfaction.

Managing Differences in Libido and Sexual Preferences

Differences in libido and sexual preferences is a usual natural phenomenon. What makes it an issue or non-issue is our attitude towards it.

Mismatched Libido:
What is libido?
A person's total sexual drive, or yearning for sexual activity, is known as libido. It is a crucial component of total well-being and affects relationships, life satisfaction, and self-worth.

There is no universally accepted level of sexual desire; everyone experiences it differently. Interest in sex can change depending on daily stressors, as well as physical and mental health.

So, what is mismatched libido?

Most relationships experience regular ups and downs, and occasionally, partners may become "stuck" on opposing sexual philosophies. When one partner has a greater libido than the other, couples experience mismatched libidos.

In relationships, mismatched libido can cause friction and result in one or both partners feeling resentful, frustrated, or inadequate. Many relationships suffer from mismatched libidos, but with patience, understanding, and safe communication, partners can work out a plan for satisfying, healthy sexual intimacy that benefits everyone.

This could entail looking for ways to make concessions, like compromising on the frequency of sex or investigating non-sexual forms of closeness. Seeking assistance from a therapist can also be beneficial as they can assist couples in resolving mismatched libido-related problems and developing coping mechanisms.

What might cause a difference in libido?

There are several reasons why two people might have mismatched libidos in a relationship. Some of the common causes are as follows:

Stress or anxiety: A person may find it difficult to feel sexual desire if they are under stress or anxiety. It may also result in other issues, such as difficulties getting lubricated or getting an erection.

Changes in hormones: A person's libido may be impacted by hormonal changes, such as those that take place during menopause or pregnancy.

Relationship problems: A couple's desire for intimacy may be impacted if they are having issues in their relationship.

Differences in sexual preferences: Different people may have different levels of sexual desire and different preferences for the kind, frequency, and location of their sex.

Changes in plans or levels of energy: An individual's need for closeness could be impacted by extreme fatigue or busyness.

Illnesses or medications: Certain medical conditions, like depression or low testosterone, can affect libido. A few medications, such as blood pressure medications or antidepressants, can also lower libido.

How can mismatched libido be improved?
It's critical that partners discuss their needs and desires in an honest and open manner, and that they look for solutions to any problems arising from mismatched libidos. There are a few things you can do to help your relationship work better if you and your partner have different libidos:

Be honest and transparent in your communication: Discuss your needs and feelings with your partner, and pay attention to their viewpoint as well. It's critical to try to reach a compromise that benefits both of you and to show empathy and respect for one another's feelings.

Look into strategies to improve intimacy: Immaturity does not always indicate the end of intimacy in a partnership. Intimacy can be increased in a variety of non-sexual ways, like holding hands, kissing, or cuddling.

Try out different approaches to intimacy: Rekindling desire can be achieved by experimenting with new activities, such as trying out different positions or introducing toys or other intimacy tools.

Allocate time for personal relationships: It's crucial to schedule intimacy time despite your hectic schedules. Making time for intimacy a priority can help guarantee that both partners are content.

Think about the impact of drugs or health issues: If one partner's libido is being negatively impacted by medication, they should consider talking to their doctor about changing the medication or changing the dosage. In a similar vein, treating a medical condition that is contributing to low libido may help increase desire.

Healing from Past Sexual Trauma or Relationship Wounds

Recovering from past relationships or sexual trauma is a very personal and frequently difficult process. The following actions can be taken by people to aid in their healing process:

Ask for Expert Assistance: Think about getting help from a counselor, therapist, or support group that specializes in trauma and recovery. A qualified expert can offer direction, affirmation, and resources to aid in navigating the healing process.

Make Self-Compassion a Practice: As you work through the healing process, treat yourself with kindness and patience. Recognize and respect your emotions, past encounters, and personal space without condemnation or guilt.

Establish Safe Areas: Be in the company of understanding and encouraging people who respect your personal space and give you a safe place to express yourself without worrying about criticism or judgment.

Establish Limits: To safeguard your mental and physical health, set up boundaries in your relationships and interactions. Advocate for your needs and assertively communicate your boundaries.

Examine Healing Approaches: To help process and release trauma stored in the body, investigate different healing modalities like mindfulness, meditation, yoga, art therapy, or somatic experiencing.

Take Care of Yourself: Make self-care activities that feed your body, mind, and spirit a priority. This can involve doing things that make you happy and fulfilled, exercising, eating well, getting enough sleep, practicing relaxation techniques, and so on.

Dispute False Beliefs: Reframe and question self-perceptions or negative beliefs that have grown out of relationship wounds or past trauma. Develop self-acceptance, self-love, and self-compassion.

Form Healthful Relationships: Assist yourself and others around you with loving, caring relationships that encourage recovery and development. Make relationships with people who honor your limits, believe in what you've gone through, and encourage you on your path to recovery.

Appreciate progress: No matter how little your progress is, acknowledge it. Honor your resiliency and strength while acknowledging the steps you've taken toward healing.

Continue to Follow Your Faith: Take solace and fortitude from your spiritual or religious convictions. Take part in activities that will help you find meaning, purpose, and connection on your path to recovery.

Seeking support and guidance along the way is acceptable because healing is a gradual and nonlinear process. Regaining a sense of empowerment and wholeness in your life after experiencing past relationships or sexual trauma is achievable with perseverance, self-compassion, and support.

Chapter Four
Cultivating Emotional and Physical Connection

In this chapter, we examine the foundations of emotional and physical intimacy in marriage. We look at the interactions between closeness and intimacy and offer practical tips and strategies for developing these important aspects of relationships. Join us as we navigate the obstacles of establishing a physical and emotional bond, empowering partners to fortify their bond and elevate their overall level of marital contentment.

Strengthening Emotional Bonds Outside of the Bedroom

It is indisputable that sexual satisfaction and relationship satisfaction are strongly correlated because humans are hardwired to use moments of physical pleasure to form close relationships with their partners. The majority of us find that physical intimacy strengthens our emotional and psychological bonding mechanisms by fostering a sense of security. In addition to strengthening attachment, this helps to further meet our needs and give us a sense of being cared for, wanted, and desired.

Even though having sex is practically the most private experience you can have with someone else, you can perform the act without really connecting at all. On the other hand, if you're only connecting in the bedroom, it might indicate that you two need to engage in other activities to develop a more intimate, emotionally charged relationship.

Humans are naturally drawn to variety, adventure, and surprise. However, regularity can occasionally negate variation, and stability is the antithesis of spontaneity. The everyday obligations of life can easily divert attention, and intimacy can suffer as a result.

Bringing intimacy outside the bedroom can be a low-key approach to enhancing our relationships' sense of fulfillment and connection. Strengthening bonds requires work; it's a process that calls for eagerness, open communication, and desire.

Activities to help you bond even when you're not in bed:
Be deliberate and sincere in your quest for better sex in your relationship.

Be Sensitive: Touch is one of the simplest ways to express intimacy; picture quick strokes, tender kisses, and even a body rub. Developing close physical proximity through mutual touching and embracing is crucial for bolstering close relationships. Touching fosters a deeper connection by gradually increasing trust between partners. Not every physical interaction needs to result in an intense makeout session. Try giving gentle kisses, holding hands more frequently, or cuddling more. To maintain romance at the forefront of our daily lives, we must cultivate a culture of touch.

Jot down a note: Writing has always been one of the finest mediums for expressing private and sensitive emotions. Receiving a handwritten note is a sentimental and romantic gesture. If that's not your thing, though, you can always text on the spur of the moment and get technical. According to research, sending flirtatious or romantic messages can make it more likely that you will pursue more personal discussions with your partners in person.

Take a Bath: According to studies, intimacy can be fostered by any kind of calming activity that calms our bodies and minds. Cuddling, back rubs, and alone or shared bath time can all become highly motivating preludes to increased intimacy and/or sex. According to reports, people will experience and desire physical intimacy in very different ways at each level of development. Even something as easy as giving your significant other a bath can spark impromptu romantic moments.

Show Love: Finding out your partner's and your love languages is another way to show and receive affection. Understanding each other's preferred interpretations of romance and love will help you communicate with your partners in a way that will deepen your relationship.

Give each other praise: Even though we frequently forget to give our partners compliments, everyone enjoys receiving them. According to studies, verbalizing compliments and displaying affection regularly can boost sensuality. We might be too preoccupied, forgetful, or preoccupied with other things. Whatever the situation, strengthening your relationship is well worth the effort.

Play around: Playful and flirtatious behavior usually comes naturally to newly formed relationships and leads to more intimate moments. It's crucial to maintain this same spirit of playfulness as relationships move into the long term to keep us bonded. Try surprising each other with a kiss or a touch to lighten the mood.

Discuss it: The best way to increase intimacy with your partners is to have sincere conversations with them. Discuss your desires for increased touch, foreplay, and connection. Couples seldom ever reach a point where they are both secure and at ease enough to discuss their fantasies. All people have desires, and discussing them with your partner can strengthen your bond.

Try taking a seat outside the bedroom and talking about your desires. When it comes to getting down to business, communication is not only critical for the relationship but also for feeling heard and understood. If you are sincere in these discussions, you can find greater fulfillment and satisfaction.

Get away: Plan an afternoon or an evening escape that will be enjoyable for both you and your partners, if only for a short while. Together, you can create experiences that strengthen your bond and promote mental clarity and relaxation. Make the most of your time apart by having uplifting, enjoyable talks that will strengthen your bonds. We frequently get into stale routines and habits, but if we're open to developing fresh experiences as a couple, breaking the mold can result in a revitalized sense of closeness.

Fostering Physical Affection and Touch

Improving physical touch and affection is a crucial part of developing intimacy and a stronger emotional bond in a relationship. The following are some strategies to develop and maintain physical affection:

Prioritize making physical contact: Do everything in your power to make regular physical contact with your spouse. This can be showing each other affection all day long through hugs, kisses, holding hands, or other tender gestures.

Show affection verbally: Talk to your partner about how much you love and appreciate them. Remind them of your love and gratitude, and let them know how much you admire the qualities in them.

Create Rituals of Attachment: Create routines or rituals that entail showing each other physical affection, like hugging each other and kissing when you get home, or spending time together before bed. These customs can support the maintenance of intimate and connected feelings.

Pay Attention and Be Present: Be present in the moment when showing your partner physical affection. Instead of allowing your thoughts to wander, concentrate on the feel of the touch and the emotional bond you have with each other.

Explore Sensual Touch: Try varying the touches and sensations until both partners find something they enjoy. To increase arousal and intimacy, this might entail giving and receiving soft touches, massages, or exploring erogenous zones.

Initiate Physical Intimacy: Make the first move to bring your partner closer to you physically. Tell them you want to touch and caress them and let them know you're open to their advances.

Express Your Preferences and Limitations: When it comes to physical affection, express your boundaries and preferences honestly and openly. Recognize your partner's comfort zone and be prepared to modify your strategy as necessary.

Arrange to Spend Quality Time Together: In your relationship, set aside specific time for physical closeness and affection. This could be organizing romantic evenings, weekend trips, or just spending time together at home.

Offer physical support: In moments of stress or emotional turmoil, provide your partner with physical support and consolation. This could be being physically there to support them, giving them a consoling touch, or just being close by.

Celebrate Physical Connection: Acknowledge and cherish the times when you and your partner experience physical closeness and intimacy. Thank God for the happiness and contentment that physical touch brings to your relationship.

You can improve intimacy, strengthen your bond, and increase emotional connection with your partner by making physical touch and affection a priority in your relationship.

Prioritizing Quality Time Together to Deepen Connection

Setting aside time for quality time together is crucial to a relationship's development of intimacy and emotional closeness. The following techniques will assist you in making time for your partner a priority:

Arrange recurring date nights: Establish a specific time each week for date nights when you can ignore all other distractions and concentrate only on each other. Make the most of this time to spend together, whether it's watching a movie at home, going out to supper, or going for a stroll in the park.

Have Intriguing Conversations: Make the most of your time together by having deep talks about subjects that are not commonly discussed. Talk to each other about your ideas, goals, and dreams, and pay attention to what your partner has to say.

Cut Off Your Technology Use: Try your best to avoid using technology when you spend quality time with each other. Make a tech-free space where you can concentrate entirely on each other by putting your phones away and turning off the TV.

Take Up New Exercises With Each Other: Take up new interests or pastimes together to keep your bond vibrant and new. Engaging in novel experiences together, such as learning to cook, traveling for a weekend, or taking up a new sport, can strengthen your bond.

Express gratitude and affection: Make the most of your time spent together by expressing your love and gratitude to your spouse. Take the time to show them love and affection and express your gratitude for all that they do, no matter how small.

Establish Traditions and Rituals: Create customs or rituals that have personal meaning for you both to help cement your relationship. This could be as easy as spending a Sunday night meal together or going on an annual trip to your preferred location.

Make Active Listening a Practice: During your time together, engage in active listening by paying close attention to what your partner is saying without any interruptions or distractions. Acknowledge their emotions and experiences while demonstrating compassion and comprehension.

Pay Attention to the Present: Keep your focus on the here and now when you're spending quality time together. Put your worries and conflicts aside so you can focus on developing your relationship and spending quality time with each other.

Unexpected gestures: To add even more specialness to your quality time together, surprise your partner with kind gestures or surprises. Little acts of kindness, like organizing a romantic picnic in the park or writing notes of love all over the house, can make a big difference in deepening your relationship.

Schedule Time for intimacy: Make physical intimacy a priority when spending quality time together to strengthen your emotional bond and keep your sexual relationship strong. To maintain the spark in your relationship, make time for tender touches, cuddles, and private times.

Setting aside time for quality time with your partner can help you both feel more emotionally connected, build your relationship, and make enduring memories.

Chapter Five

Reigniting Passion and Rediscovering Desire

Let's look at the process of reviving passion and desire in a married relationship. We look at ways to lighten the intimacy and spark again in the relationship through doable tactics and perceptive advice. Come along on this self-discovery with us as we help couples rediscover the depth of their desire for a more vibrant and satisfying marital bond and to rekindle their passion.

Exploring Sexual Fantasies and New Experiences Together

Having new experiences together is a thrilling and personal journey that can strengthen a couple's bond and increase their level of sexual satisfaction. Stepping outside of one's comfort zone, being honest about one's goals and boundaries, and adopting an adventurous and curious mindset are all necessary for this exploration.

Establishing a secure and accepting environment for candid conversation is one of the first steps toward investigating sexual fantasies and novel experiences together. This entails making time for open discussions about fantasies, boundaries, and desires without worrying about being judged or criticized. It's critical that both partners feel free to communicate their wants and needs and that they will be acknowledged and listened to.

Couples can start experimenting with new experiences and exploring various avenues to realize their fantasies once they have established communication. This could entail exploring role-playing scenarios or it could entail experimenting with various sexual activities, positions, or techniques. It's important to approach these encounters with an open mind and a desire to jointly try new things.

Prioritizing mutual consent and respect is crucial for couples venturing into new sexual experiences and fantasies. This calls for frequent check-ins, respect for one another's personal space, and a readiness to change course or stop if something bothers you or goes too far. It's crucial to keep in mind that fantasies are precisely that, fantasies, and that not all of them must be realized in the actual world. Sometimes all it takes to increase arousal and intimacy between partners is to simply talk about fantasies.

Couples can gain from experimenting in the bedroom and broadening their sexual horizons in addition to delving into their fantasies and novel experiences. This could entail incorporating sex toys or props or experimenting with various forms of touch. It's important to approach these interactions with curiosity and playfulness and to concentrate on finding mutual enjoyment and fulfillment.

How to Get Better at Sex More Frequently

Clearly state your intentions: Effective communication is essential to increasing both the quantity and quality of your sex. It's critical to express your needs in the relationship in a general way since effective communication fosters trust and maintains a healthy partnership. However, it is also crucial that you let your partner know what you need in terms of sex.

Teach your partner how to please you: Teach your partner how to please you if they're not doing it exactly right. Helping someone who seems awkward or even like you might be hurting their feelings is ultimately what they're trying to do for you. In addition, respect your partner's direct communication and follow their instructions if they are given to you.

Do your part: You should communicate your desires to your partner, but you shouldn't put all the pressure on them to comply! To be able to communicate your own sexual needs to your partner, you must first be aware of them. Consequently, it's also essential to wake yourself up when needed.

Acknowledge your Passions: Even though your partner is the most attractive person on the planet, they may not be able to arouse or make you feel good all by themselves. Acknowledge your passions and occasionally offer assistance. It's seductive to know what you want, and your partner will appreciate any guidance that makes you enjoy yourself more during sex.

Plan some quality time for you two: Intimacy is frequently the first thing to go when life becomes too much to handle. If you're overly stressed out and have a million things on your plate, it can be difficult to feel wantable or think about having sex. However, neglecting intimacy and sexual relations during periods of stress can seriously harm your partnership. Even when you think you won't be able to fit anything more into your day, it's crucial to maintain a close relationship with your spouse. Making plans for quality time spent together can help to guarantee that your sex life isn't neglected when things get tough.

Sexual Schedule: When you're completely frustrated, having a sexual schedule can also provide you with something to look forward to! Play into that by scheduling things well in advance. A lot of the pleasure of having sex is the build-up to it and the thoughts that follow. In keeping with this, it can also be enjoyable to arrange a brief vacation where you can concentrate solely on spending quality time with your significant other. Rent a hotel room, or even organize a camping trip where the only thing on the schedule is quality time spent together.

Remove it from the sleeping area: While setting aside time in your calendar to guarantee that you spend some quality time together can be beneficial, don't underestimate the allure of spontaneity! Even though we make a lot of effort to regulate our feelings and other aspects of our lives, there are moments when sexual desire overcomes us. It's not necessary for sex to be limited to the kind of romantic bedroom scenes we see in movies.

Making the most of your sex drive when and where it arises can result in incredibly thrilling interactions. Having sex somewhere other than the bedroom can add spontaneity and fun to your sexual life. You name it: showers, couches, and countertops. While it's not necessary to completely banish sex from the house, maintaining discretion and being inventive can spice up your relationship.

Put intimacy before sex: If you want more sex, that's great, but you shouldn't devote all of your energy to it. If you or your partner are nervous about having sex or experience performance anxiety, focusing on sex can be daunting and even overwhelming. Rather, concentrate on developing closeness. This can be achieved by taking a break from sexual activity to concentrate on physical intimacy-building activities like kissing and hugs, which will develop physical intimacy without necessarily leading to sex. Interactions that don't involve sexual activity but still require touch, like messaging, can also promote intimacy. When the break ends, doing this can enhance your emotional bond and lead to better, more intimate sex.

Take your time during foreplay: Even though everyone enjoys a good quickie, it's crucial that not every moment of your sex is brief and direct. Then again, one of the most enjoyable aspects of sex can be foreplay. Increasing the duration of foreplay can enhance the anticipation of having sex and improve its overall enjoyment. Regardless of whether you are "giving" or "receiving" pleasure, foreplay is enjoyable. It's a method of making your sex more intimate by including kissing, caressing, and all the other good stuff. Playful sex can also result from foreplay. Great sex can also result from teasing and other similar activities during your foreplay. It's not necessary for sex to always be pure passion.

Try out different roles: Your close relationship may take on a delightful new dimension through experimentation. Finding new positions will improve your sex and keep things interesting, even though not every new position will work out!

Don't hesitate to take the lead: It's crucial to alternate who initiates sexual contact. Sensing that your partner wants you is a crucial component of having sex, and the main way to express your desire is to initiate intimacy and sex. It's simple to get into a routine where one person always starts the conversation, but switching things up will demonstrate to both partners their sexual desirability. Altering the person who initiates can also inspire more imaginative sexual behavior; altering the initiation patterns can lead to

Introducing Variety and Spontaneity into Your Sexual Relationship Maintaining a healthy sexual life can occasionally be challenging in a committed, long-term relationship. Even if you're still completely smitten with your partner, it's easy for things to go a bit dull in the bedroom once those first butterflies pass and you get used to your regular routines. Thankfully, there are always ways to liven up your sexual life, no matter what your sex preferences.

Spanking:
Spanking is another sexy and entertaining way to add some kink to your bedroom situation, as long as the other person has given their consent.

Take a holiday:
Vacations are beneficial, particularly for individuals who have kids or are in committed relationships. You can become sufficiently relaxed to feel sexually at ease by leaving your area, where you don't have to clean, or by ordering room service. To put it briefly, interruptions and ensuring that everything is tidy afterward are not concerns.

Engage in some sexual gaming:
Something that adds something fresh to your sexual life? Games are great, especially the more free-form ones like playing cards or dice.

Begin texting while you're not around: Your sex life will be spiced up perfectly with kinky and dirty messages. Send messages along the lines of "I can't wait to suck your nipples" or "I want you to suck me when you get home."

It's a method of preparing for and creating anticipation for sex. That excitement is already there when they get home. In essence, ratcheting up the sexual tension throughout the day signals to your partner that they are the object of your affection and gets you both excited.

You can always choose to role-play:
Consider adding some role-playing to your sex life to spice it up. For those who are unsure of where to start, a romantic dinner is a great option. Take advantage of the opportunity to connect by going on a date, but act as though it's your first time meeting. Anticipation will mount as you get ready to meet, which adds a little spice to the relationship.

As you would "get ready" for a date, tell your partner to "pick you up" at a specific time and put on an outfit that gives you confidence. When the time comes for you to return home, you can continue the act as though it's your first time sleeping together.

Create a playlist for sex:
Play your preferred soundtrack and enjoy a sexual encounter while it plays. Make a fun playlist together and add songs that give you both a sense of empowerment, comfort, and most importantly, arousal.

Include food in the mixture:
Nothing says sweetness quite like sex play that includes chocolate, whipped cream, and/or strawberries. Try feeding each other, licking the components off of each other, or even making amusing phallic gestures with the food. You can make it as lighthearted and enjoyable as you like.

Get a few sexy underwear:
Since humans are primarily visual beings, lingerie can even help you feel more at ease in your skin, enabling you to engage in sexual activity and be seen. It can, in essence, be a really powerful confidence booster.

Admit your true emotions:
Perhaps becoming more in tune with your true feelings about the act as a whole is necessary to spice up your sex life. Speak with a professional if you're experiencing uncomfortable feelings during sex or anxiety before engaging in it.

This is particularly true if you believe that trauma may be the cause of these reactions. It is unrealistic to expect your partner to take care of you, so get in touch with those medical professionals. After discussing your feelings with your partner, devise a plan that involves having sex that you find enjoyable and relaxing.

Have sex to makeup:
Many people find that they can rekindle their relationship through makeup sex after a fight or other stressful situations. After a heated dispute, getting together is great because you're venting your frustrations on each other, but make sure you deal with the underlying issue. Although it shouldn't be seen as a panacea for relationship problems, having sex can benefit both you and your partner.

Overcoming Monotony and Routine in the Bedroom

You must abandon routine and monotony in the bedroom if you want to preserve passion and excitement in your sexual relationship. To help you keep the spark alive and spice things up, consider the following strategies:

Communicate Openly: Talk to your partner about the fantasies, desires, and experiences you hope to have in the bedroom. In addition, encourage them to be willing to try new things and to express their own desires.

Do New Things: To mix up your daily routine, try experimenting with different sexual positions, activities, and strategies. Keep an open mind and be willing to step outside of your comfort zone.

Show Your Variability: Incorporate some diversity into your sexual life to shake things up. Try varying the locations, times of day, or even role-playing scenarios to add some spice to your sexual life.

Utilize Sensory Information: Make use of all your senses during sex to enhance pleasure and arousal. Try using silk sheets, sensual music, or scented candles to create a sensual atmosphere in your bedroom.

Include Playthings and Accessory Items: Use sex toys, lingerie, or other accessories to spice up your romantic encounters with excitement and exploration. To improve enjoyment for all involved, be open to trying out novel techniques and equipment.

Pay attention Foreplay: Spend more time in foreplay to heighten arousal and anticipation prior to sexual activity. Try different methods of caressing, kissing, and touching to increase intimacy and pleasure.

Indulge in fantasy: Together, explore your sexual fantasies and come up with ways to fulfill them in bed. Playing role-playing games, watching sensuous movies, and engaging in erotic storytelling can all spark creativity and passion.

Set Up Sexual Dates: Make time on your calendar for personal interactions and set priorities for them. This can ensure that you consistently carve out time for one another and prevent sex from becoming a secondary priority.

Prioritize connecting with others: Focus on strengthening your physical and emotional bond with your partner during sex. Be open-minded, loving, and truthful in your communication throughout the interaction.

Celebrate Accomplishment: Respect your attempts to escape monotony and routine in the bedroom, no matter how small. Respect and honor each other's openness to trying new things if you want to keep the spark in your relationship alive.

By employing these strategies, you can keep the spark alive in the bedroom for years to come without becoming stale or bored. Remember that open communication and a willingness to explore are necessary for having a happy and fulfilling sexual life with your partner.

Chapter Six

Embracing Change and Growth in Your Sexual Relationship

We explore the process of accepting change and development in your sexual relationship in this chapter. Understanding that all lasting relationships must evolve, we look into the chances that come with accepting change to strengthen intimacy and connection. Let's go through the challenges of this reality, enabling couples to develop a more satisfying and exciting sexual relationship through mutual development, openness, and adaptation.

Accepting the Evolution of Your Sexual Connection

Keeping a happy and healthy relationship over time requires you to accept how your sexual connection changes over time. As a seasoned professional, I've seen firsthand how couples deal with the alterations in their sexual dynamics that come with time.

Understand that every long-term relationship, including the sexual component, will inevitably undergo change. Couples' dynamics change and grow together, just like people do. The first step to embracing the evolution of your sexual connection is acknowledging this reality. Your sexual connection may go through several phases as time goes on, depending on things like stressors, life events, and personal development. Accept the variety of experiences that come with being in a committed relationship and keep an open mind when it comes to discovering new, deep ways to bond with your spouse.

Going through changes in your sexual connection requires effective communication. Establish a judgment-free, safe space where you and your partner can talk freely about your desires, thoughts, feelings, and worries related to your sexual relationship. You can encourage a deeper understanding and connection by talking about your experiences and listening to each other with empathy.

Give priority to the quality of your intimate moments rather than just the quantity of sex. The degree of emotional connection, mutual satisfaction, and pleasure felt by both partners can be used to gauge quality. You and your partner can develop a more fulfilling and meaningful sexual relationship if you put quality above quantity. As one another's needs and preferences change, be accommodating and flexible with one another. Your tastes, priorities, and physical capacities may change over time as individuals and as a couple. Accept these changes with an open mind and a desire to discover new things as a team.

Realize that emotional intimacy and connection are just as important to a sexual relationship as physical acts. A fulfilling sexual relationship requires emotional intimacy, vulnerability, and understanding, so cultivate these moments with your partner. See a therapist or counselor who specializes in sexual health and intimacy if you are having trouble navigating the changes in your sexual connection on your own. A qualified expert can offer direction, insight, and resources to support you in making this journey gracefully and empathetically.

It takes honesty, communication, flexibility, and a dedication to developing closeness and connection with your partner to embrace the evolution of your sexual relationship. You can develop a long-lasting and satisfying sexual relationship by accepting the changes that occur with time and upholding a strong emotional bond.

Communicating Changing Needs and Desires

To keep your relationship happy and healthy, you both need to communicate your evolving needs and desires. Here's how to approach this conversation with the professionalism of an experienced party:

Establish a Secure and Helpful Environment: Begin by establishing a secure and encouraging space where you and your spouse can freely and honestly express yourselves. Pick a time for this crucial task that will allow you to both be at ease and unhindered.

Make Use of "I" Statements: Without assigning blame or making accusations, use "I" statements to frame your communication and express your own needs, wants, and feelings. Rather than uttering, "You never satisfy me anymore," for instance, consider expressing, "I've been feeling a bit disconnected lately, and I'd like to explore ways to reignite our intimacy."

Be Particular and Detailed: Clearly state any new interests or preferences you've developed, as well as any specific changes you've noticed in your needs and desires. Giving specific examples can make it easier for your partner to understand your perspective and how they can assist you.

Promote Intense Listening: Urge your companion to pay attention to what you're saying without interrupting or making snap judgments. As you converse with them, practice empathy and understanding and let them respond with their thoughts and feelings.

Pay Attention to Solutions: Take a cooperative approach to the discussion, concentrating on coming to agreements and solutions that benefit you both. Discuss ways to accommodate one another's evolving needs and preferences while preserving a solid and wholesome relationship.

Be Receptive to Input: Remain receptive to your partner's input regarding their evolving needs and preferences. It's crucial to keep in mind that communication is two-way and to pay attention to and respect their experiences as well.

Assure Your Companion: Assure your partner that their inadequacy or failure is not reflected in your changing needs and desires. Reaffirm your love and dedication for them, and make it clear that the goal of this talk is to improve your bond and strengthen your relationship.

Have Reasonable Expectations: Recognize that change takes time, and it's acceptable if you and your spouse don't immediately know the answers. As you work through this process together, set reasonable expectations for yourselves and show each other patience and support.

Continue as Before: Regularly check in with each other to discuss any new developments or concerns that may come up, as well as to find out how you're both feeling about the progress you've made. A solid and healthy relationship requires constant and open communication.

You may successfully communicate your evolving needs and desires to your partner and work together to build your relationship by going into the conversation with empathy, candor, and a willingness to work together.

Embracing Challenges as Opportunities for Sexual Growth and Exploration

Developing a transformative mindset that views challenges as chances for sexual development and exploration can improve relationships and increase levels of intimacy. Reframe issues in your sexual relationship as opportunities for personal growth and exploration rather than as challenges that need to be overcome. Acknowledge that difficulties can result in increased intimacy, comprehension, and pleasure from sex with your partner.

Recognize that infidelity is a natural and inevitable aspect of any relationship. A multitude of factors, including stress, exhaustion, changes in libido, and life transitions, can impact sexual dynamics. By normalizing these difficulties, you can face them with greater acceptance and openness rather than with feelings of inadequacy or guilt.

Any problems you're having in your sexual relationship should be discussed openly and honestly with your partner. Be open and honest with your partner about your desires, emotions, and worries, and encourage them to be the same. Together, you can overcome obstacles more skillfully if you can establish a conversational environment that is safe and judgment-free.

Take advantage of obstacles to your advantage to pinpoint and investigate areas in your sexual relationship that still need work. Think of the things you want to try, the things you both enjoy doing, and the changes you want to make. As you approach this process, keep an open mind, exercise creativity, and show willingness to try new things. Never be afraid to ask for resources and assistance to help you and your partner through difficult times and enhance your sexual exploration. This can entail reading books or articles, going to seminars or workshops, consulting with a therapist or counselor who specializes in intimacy and sexual health, or doing all three.

To become more understanding and intimate with your partner, own your vulnerability. Discuss your shortcomings, fears, and insecurities with your partner in an open and sincere manner. Exposing oneself to one another can improve your relationship and promote empathy and trust. Recognize that developing and exploring one's sexuality takes time and patience. As you try new things and overcome obstacles, have patience with one another and with yourself. Never give up on your desire to explore and develop as a sexual being, and celebrate your little victories along the way.

Respect the strides you two take as you overcome obstacles and discover new ways to express your sexuality. Appreciate and respect the work you and your partner put into maintaining your sexual relationship, and relish the intimate, pleasurable, and connecting times you two share. You and your partner can grow closer, experience greater pleasure, and fortify your relationship by viewing obstacles as chances for sexual exploration and growth. Courage, open-mindedness, and readiness to delve into the depths of your sexual connection are essential as you proceed to win together.

Chapter Seven
Overcoming Common Sexual Roadblocks

Let's address the typical roadblocks that can prevent sexual fulfillment in relationships. We explore doable tactics for rekindling passion and getting past obstacles like poor communication and stage anxiety. Let's also discuss the difficulties of having a sexual relationship, giving couples the tools they need to get past obstacles and build a happier, more fulfilling union.

Managing Performance Anxiety and Sexual Dysfunction

Worries about one's expectations from one's partner and personal issues can intensify anxiety related to sexual performance. Erectile dysfunction and anxiety associated with sexual performance can be managed in a number of ways.

Sexual stress can trigger performance anxiety. This could lead to erectile dysfunction, which is the inability to get or keep an erection. Employing a few simple coping strategies can help people with erectile dysfunction brought on by performance anxiety.

What connection exists between erectile dysfunction and performance anxiety?
Erectile dysfunction and performance anxiety may be related in a number of ways. Sexual dysfunction can arise in any person, regardless of gender, due to stress and anxiety related to sexual performance or pleasing a partner.

A person may begin to feel unworthy or incapable if they are unable to live up to their partner's sexual expectations. Low self-esteem and feelings of inadequacy can result in physical symptoms like erectile dysfunction. Psychological factors are listed by researchers as one of the multiple causes of erectile dysfunction. Stated differently, an individual's mental state can impact their sexual performance.

Reasons why people get performance anxiety

When someone has unfavorable thoughts about their capacity to perform well during sexual activity, they often experience performance anxiety. An individual might be concerned about their ability to satisfy a partner or their lack of sexual adequacy. These emotions may be influenced by the following factors:

- Body image
- Penis circumference
- Views on virility
- Notions of gender roles
- Relationship problems
- Using porn on the internet

An individual's mental health may be impacted and performance anxiety may be exacerbated by revolving financial worries, family conflicts, or workplace stress.

Causes of Erectile Dysfunction

These factors may contribute to issues of erectile dysfunction:

- Hormonal equilibrium
- Neurological components
- Blood flow
- Psychological aspects and mental health
- Depression
- Apathy

- Decline in appeal
- Tension
- Low amounts of testosterone
- Cigarette use
- Misuse of drugs or alcohol
- Persistent ailments
- Kidney conditions
- Diabetic nerve damage
- Stroke
- Radiation to the pelvis
- Lately performed surgery

Several drugs, particularly those that interfere with or change hormones, nerves, or blood pressure, can also lead to erectile dysfunction. Among them are:

- Depression-fighting drugs
- Anti-inflammatory drugs
- Prescription drugs for high blood pressure
- Medications for erratic heart rhythm
- Relaxants for muscles
- Hormone replacement treatment
- Chemotherapy
- Medications that impact the prostate

Before taking a new medication, a person can get assistance from a doctor or pharmacist in identifying possible side effects.

Mental health and erectile dysfunction:

There is more to erectile dysfunction than meets the eye. It could affect someone's relationships, mental health, and social life. Researchers have found links between erectile dysfunction and anxiety, tension, depression, low self-esteem, low confidence, relationship issues, and insomnia. Performance anxiety may result from these or be its root cause.

If an individual experiences an erection upon awakening but not during sexual engagement, there might be a psychological or emotional reason. Treatment and counseling in psychology, such as cognitive behavioral therapy, can help people get over issues related to ED and sexual performance.

Signs and symptoms:

Since different people react differently to stress and anxiety, performance anxiety affects people differently. Performance anxiety may result in:

- Early ejaculation
- Incapacity to climax
- Absence of desire for sex

Additionally, studies indicate that heterosexual individuals with performance anxiety may be more inclined to pursue extramarital sex. One of the physical signs of erectile dysfunction is having trouble achieving or maintaining an erection. It might also cause one to lose their desire for sex.

How to handle Erectile dysfunction:

A variety of strategies can assist individuals in managing their ED and performance anxiety while facilitating satisfying sexual encounters.

Steer clear of the cycle:

Most people occasionally have unpleasant sexual experiences. Usually, occasional erectile dysfunction is not a reason for alarm. On the other hand, dwelling on the disappointment can prevent future sexual activity if it causes fear and anxiety, and these feelings can last. It is critical to understand that a person's occasional incapacity to perform does not imply that they are incapable of engaging in sexual activity.

It could indicate that they were experiencing tension or worry at the moment. They'll be able to enjoy sex just as much later, when the stress is gone. A person may find it easier to lessen the pressure they put on themselves to perform well every time by changing their attention from the symptoms to the cause, especially during stressful times.

Become aware of your senses:
An individual experiencing performance anxiety may constantly replay in their mind their perceived shortcomings in romantic relationships and obsess over their partner's or other partners' thoughts. It may be helpful to focus solely on the senses rather than overthinking or overanalyzing what transpired during sex.

You can avoid worrying about your performance by focusing on the feelings in your hands and the images in your eyes. Scent-filled candles and music could heighten the sensory experience while reducing anxiety.

Exercise:
Research has indicated a link between erectile dysfunction symptoms and minimal to nonexistent physical activity. Completing a simple 20–30 minute exercise routine a few times a week may be advantageous as it can enhance overall health and reduce stress.

Other methods:
- Erectile dysfunction and performance anxiety can be treated with a variety of other methods. Among them are:
- Guided breathing exercises, like
- Therapy using guided imagery
- Couples therapy
- Sexual counseling
- Stress-relieving techniques like yoga and mindfulness
- Quitting porn and masturbating

Being honest about one's feelings of performance anxiety with any potential sexual partners may also be beneficial. By doing this, the partner can assist the person in finding ways to cope with their anxiety and help them feel less stressed.

When to visit a physician:
Medical treatment may be helpful if lifestyle changes and relaxation methods do not alleviate symptoms, or if symptoms worsen over time. A physician can provide guidance on other treatment options, such as combining medication and psychotherapy.

Handling Differences in Sexual Appetite and Preferences

An essential element of close relationships, sexual desire is as individual as the people involved. However, what occurs when a partner's flame of desire burns differently?

For clarity, waning of sexual desire doesn't translate to waning of love and affection. Also discrepancy in sexual appetite and preferences doesn't mean lack of affection. Muddling the two up causes more misunderstanding.

Understanding Desire Discrepancies
When one person in a relationship has a higher or lower libido than the other, it can lead to desire disparities. While a certain amount of desire fluctuates over time, major changes can present difficulties. These differences have a multitude of underlying causes:

Biological Factors: A number of biological, hormonal, and genetic factors affect our libidos. Divergent sexual appetites may result from differences in these factors.

Psychological Factors: A person's desire for sex can be greatly impacted by stress, anxiety, depression, traumatic experiences in the past, or problems with body image.

Relationship Dynamics: A person's degree of sexual desire is significantly influenced by their overall health and their current romantic situation. Inequality can be caused by persistent disagreements, poor communication, or emotional disengagement.

Life Transitions: One's sexual desire may change as a result of significant life events such as becoming a parent, changing careers, aging, or health problems.

Addressing Desire Discrepancies

Resolving desire disparities requires open, sincere, and compassionate communication. Here's how to overcome this typical obstacle in relationships:

Start the conversation: Locate a private, safe, and quiet area where you can talk about your desires. When addressing the subject, take your partner's or partners' feelings into account.

Listen attentively: Regardless of disagreements, always keep in mind that your partner(s)' desires are just as valid as yours. Pay close attention to what they have to say without jumping in or making judgments right away.

Determine the Primary Reasons: Look into the underlying causes of the variations in desire. Are there any other factors, like stress or unresolved interpersonal disputes? The first step in solving a problem is identifying its underlying cause.

Set Reasonably High Bars: Understand that in any relationship, your sexual desires will change. Experiencing different levels of desire is common.

Make a compromise: Perhaps a compromise is the best way to address this issue. Achieving a fair balance may require one or more partners to make sacrifices.

Ask Professional Advice: It could be a good idea to speak with a therapist or counselor who specializes in relationship and sexual issues if you are experiencing notable fluctuations in your desire.

Enhancing Intimacy Beyond Sex

Although it's a vital component of romantic relationships, intimacy can take other forms besides sexual desire. Increasing emotional closeness, connection, and trust can also help to fortify the relationship between partners. The following are some tactics:

Spending Quality Time: Take some time to relax outside of bed. Take part in things you both like to do to establish a deeper connection.

Skillful Interaction: To promote emotional intimacy, work on your communication abilities. Talk about your feelings, ideas, and fears.

Fondness: Even when there are differences in sexual desire, physical affection such as cuddling, kissing, and hugging can help sustain a sense of closeness.

Astonishment and Instinct: Surprise your partner and add spontaneity to your daily routine to keep your relationship lively.

Investigate Together: Aim for novel experiences in and out of the bedroom to maintain the spark and excitement in your relationship.

Help for Therapy: Sex therapy or couples therapy can offer a secure setting for discussing differences in desire and developing intimacy-enhancing techniques.

Different sexual desires are a frequent source of conflict in many partnerships. They don't have to, however, be a cause of strife or disagreement. In a relationship, it is crucial that partners feel heard, respected, and valued in both private and public settings. Every relationship is different.

Seeking Professional Support and Guidance When Needed

It is proactive and empowering to seek professional support and guidance when needed to address issues and improve sexual well-being in a relationship. This is why it matters, along with some guidance on how to deal with it:

Establishing Assistance Requests as Normal: Recognize that seeking professional assistance for sex-related problems is typical and expected. As with all facets of health and wellness, sexual health is something that requires consideration and maintenance. Seeking assistance indicates that you place a high value on the health and happiness of your partnership.

Complete Information: Recognize the expertise and experience sexual health professionals, such as counselors, therapists, or sex therapists, have in addressing sexual issues and advancing sexual health. They can offer perceptive guidance, practical resources, and solutions tailored to your particular circumstance.

A Safe and Confidential Environment: With expert assistance, you and your spouse can discuss your concerns, feelings, desires, and challenges openly without fear of stigma or condemnation. Real progress and development are made possible by the atmosphere's encouragement of empathy, understanding, and trust.

Detailed Analysis: Your sexual health concerns can be thoroughly assessed by a specialist in the field, who will consider your personal history, relationship dynamics, psychological well-being, and physical health. This holistic approach makes it possible to fully comprehend the issues at hand and to plan treatments with knowledge.

Empirically Based Interventions: Sexual health professionals use evidence-based interventions and therapeutic techniques to address a wide range of sexual concerns, including communication issues, desire discrepancies, performance anxiety, trauma recovery, and intimacy enhancement. Because they are tailored to your specific needs and goals, these interventions promote effective and durable results.

Empowerment and Skill Development: You and your partner can overcome obstacles in your sexual life and enhance your sexual well-being on your own with the assistance of a professional. Behavioral interventions, practice speaking with others, and education can all help you become more resilient, self-aware, and confident in your ability to handle sexual concerns.

Counseling for couples and duals: Depending on your needs and goals, therapy sessions can be either individual, couple, or combination. Individual therapy may address personal problems or issues that impact one's sexual health, while couples therapy seeks to improve communication, resolve conflicts, and strengthen the partnership.

Continuous Support and Monitoring: In order to monitor progress, address new problems, and reinforce positive changes, professional assistance typically involves ongoing supervision and follow-up, rather than just one session. With this ongoing assistance, your sexual relationship will progressively expand and deepen over time.

To sum up, you can resolve sexual issues, promote intimacy, and advance sexual well-being in your relationship by proactively seeking out professional support and guidance when needed. You can overcome challenges, create a fulfilling relationship, and feel more connected and content with your partner if you prioritize your sexual health and seek professional help.

Chapter Eight

Sustaining Long-Term Sexual Satisfaction

Let's look at the key tactics that will help you maintain long-term sexual satisfaction in your partnership. To guarantee long-lasting fulfillment, we explore useful insights and doable actions on everything from preserving intimacy to overcoming obstacles. Come along as we explore the challenges of maintaining a satisfying sexual relationship, giving couples the tools they need to build a remarkably fulfilling and long-lasting bond.

Committing to Continuous sexual Improvement and Exploration

Deepening intimacy, satisfaction, and connection in your relationship by resolving to pursue ongoing sexual growth and exploration. This is a lively and fruitful journey. Take a growth-oriented approach, considering sexual intimacy as a process of learning and growth rather than a destination. It will be easier for you to accept the idea that there's always room for development and new experiences if you approach the study of sexuality with an open mind, curiosity, and willingness to learn new skills.

Encourage the open and honest discussion of your sexual preferences, fantasies, desires, and concerns with your partner. Regularly discuss what is going well and what could be better. Examine methods together for improving your sex life. Establish goals for exploring and improving your sexuality that both of you can agree upon and that take into consideration the needs and preferences of your partners. These objectives could be anything from exploring novel methods or postures to growing closeness and emotional connection. To monitor your progress and recognize your accomplishments along the way, set measurable goals and benchmarks.

Aim to become knowledgeable about intimacy, pleasure, and sexual health. To learn more about sexual wellness and improve your knowledge and abilities, read books, articles, and reliable resources. You can also go to seminars or workshops and get advice from professionals in the field. Experiment with different approaches, experiences, and sexual activities to keep your relationship fresh, exciting, and fulfilling. As a couple, be open to trying new activities like role-playing, utilizing sex toys, or experimenting with sensual massage techniques.

Prioritize your partner's happiness and fulfillment throughout your sexual encounters. Take equal time to become acquainted with one another's bodies, erogenous zones, and preferences. Happiness is something that you ought to value equally on both sides. Talk openly about what feels and doesn't, and be mindful of each other's needs and cues. You can develop presence and mindfulness by focusing entirely on your sex. Try practicing relaxation techniques, sensory awareness, and deep breathing exercises to enhance your enjoyment and your relationship with your partner.

Celebrate each and every advancement you two have made in your sexual journey, no matter how tiny. Treasure the times you get to spend together experiencing pleasure, intimacy, and closeness, and respect the efforts you both put in to strengthen your sexual bond. If you run into issues or obstacles while exploring your sexuality, get professional help. Counselors, therapists, and sex therapists can help you overcome obstacles and fulfill your sexual desires. They can also provide information, support, and guidance.

Remain committed to consistent, long-term sexual growth and exploration. Maintain your commitment to growing your sexual relationship with your partner and see failures or challenges as opportunities for growth. By making a commitment to continuous sexual development and exploration, you and your partner can create a profound, meaningful, and incredibly fulfilling sexual relationship. It's possible for this relationship to change and expand over time. With an open mind, a desire to discover, and a commitment to pleasure and intimacy, set out on this adventure together.

Prioritizing Self-Care and Sexual Wellness

It is essential to prioritize sexual wellness and self-care if you want to keep yourself and your partner happy and healthy. Taking the following actions will help you prioritize your tasks like a seasoned pro:

Recognize its significance: Understand that the longevity of your relationship and your health depend on you placing a high priority on your own sexual and physical well-being. You must first invest the time and energy necessary to care for yourself if you hope to have a healthy and happy relationship with your spouse.

Clearly Defined Restrictions: To make sure you have the resources to give your sexual and self-care a high priority, set clear boundaries for your time, energy, and personal space. Set firm boundaries and assert your needs in the relationship by communicating with your partner.

Develop a Habit of Self-Care: Develop self-care as a daily habit to maintain your mental, emotional, and physical health. These include going to the gym, exercising, writing in a journal, getting outside, and taking up enjoyable hobbies.

Prioritize your sexual health above all else: Prioritize your sexual health by making time for routine doctor's appointments, engaging in safe sexual behavior, and keeping up with the most recent developments regarding STIs and contraception. To preserve general well-being, address any issues or worries related to sexual health as soon as possible.

Promote Emotional Capability: To become attuned to your feelings, desires, and boundaries regarding your sexuality, cultivate emotional awareness and mindfulness. Be kind and accepting to yourself when you experience your feelings and keep in mind your beliefs, past experiences, and moral standards around intimacy and sex.

Transparent Communication: Promote honest dialogue about your boundaries, worries, and desires regarding your sexual life with your partner. Establish a conversational environment that is secure, free of bias, and supportive of each partner's right to self-expression and sexual exploration.

Discover Contentment: Realize that engaging in safe, intimate sexual relationships requires having fun. Spend some time getting to know your body and what makes you happy, whether it's through experiences you share with your partner or time spent alone masturbating. Make sex a priority if you want to feel content, joyful, and connected.

Invest in Close Relationships: You and your partner can develop a close relationship through telling each other stories, exposing yourself emotionally, and making deep connections. Establishing and strengthening your relationship can be achieved through scheduling meaningful conversations, spending time together, and expressing your love and affection regularly.

Look for Expert Assistance: Never be afraid to consult with trained professionals if you're having problems or have questions about your sexual health or self-care. You can get the direction, encouragement, and resources you need from therapists, counselors, or sex therapists to help you deal with these circumstances with assurance and clarity.

Appreciate your milestones: Honor your path toward sexual and self-care wellness as a symbol of your dedication to your development and welfare. Continue to take good care of yourself and your relationship while acknowledging the progress, realizations, and connections you've made along the way.

You can improve your sense of fulfillment, vitality, and connection in your relationship with your partner and yourself by prioritizing your sex and self-care needs. Treat this rearranging of priorities with kindness, curiosity, and a dedication to your well-being.

Celebrating Sexual Milestones and Achievements Together

Celebrating successes together is a wonderful way to strengthen your bond, foster intimacy, and acknowledge the growth and development of your sexual relationship. Take some time to celebrate and honor the milestones and moments of sexual growth that you have shared together. To achieve this, one may need to overcome challenges, try new things, get closer, or simply enjoy private times.

Reflect on how far you two have come in your sexual relationship, both separately and together. Recall the progress you've made since the beginning of your journey and give thanks for the time, energy, and dedication you've both invested in growing your sexual partnership. In addition to their contributions to your sexual relationship, thank your partner for being a kind and encouraging travel companion. Tell them how much you appreciate their curiosity, candor, and commitment to sharing pleasure and fulfillment with you both.

Arrange special occasions or get-togethers to celebrate your shared sexual successes. A romantic dinner, a weekend getaway, a sensual massage, or anything else that allows you to connect and deeply celebrate your achievements could be examples of this. Establish rites or traditions to regularly mark significant junctures in your romantic life. This can be a monthly check-in to see how you're doing, an annual anniversary celebration, or a quarterly retreat to celebrate your journey together and reignite your relationship.

Take some time to reflect on your romantic relationship's memorable moments and interactions. Recall the happy times, amusing tales, or transformative experiences that have shaped your journey together. As proof of your relationship, cherish these memories. Don't miss this opportunity to express your love and gratitude for your spouse. Give them love, kindness, and compliments to foster and strengthen your relationship.

Make plans and goals for your sex life based on the future. Have a conversation about your goals as a couple, such as trying new things, growing closer emotionally, or finding more fulfillment and pleasure. Consider documenting your sexual journey together with journal entries, letter exchanges, or photos. Seize moments of joy, education, and camaraderie, then reflect on them collectively to assess your development and further adventures.

Mostly, just remember to live in the now and appreciate the occasion as you commemorate your shared sexual achievements. Cherish the experience as you and your companion progress and mature together, and focus on the love, closeness, and bond you have in common. By celebrating your accomplishments and sexual milestones together, you can deepen your connection, become more intimate, and develop a stronger sense of connection and appreciation for one another. Resolve to maintain a solid sexual relationship for years to come, and celebrate this occasion with gratitude and joy.

Encouragement for Readers to Apply Lessons Learned

Let's look at some ideas to help you put "Sex in Your Marriage"'s lessons into practice:

Accept the Journey: Keep in mind that increasing your marriage's intimacy and sexual satisfaction is a process rather than a destination. When you work through obstacles and put new plans into action, have patience with both yourself and your partner.

Transparent Communication: Make a commitment to communicating your needs, wants, and worries to your partner in an honest and open manner. Establish a conversational environment where you both feel supported, heard, and understood.

Move Forward: Don't just read the book; apply the ideas and tactics it offers. Put the advice to use, try out some new strategies, and observe which ones suit your relationship the best.

Appreciate the Progress: Enjoy each and every victory and advancement in your sex life. Acknowledge the efforts you and your partner are making to strengthen your bond and express gratitude to one another for your mutual commitment to self-improvement.

Seek Assistance: Never be embarrassed to seek the advice of professionals when you need more guidance or encounter difficulties. You can get specialized advice and resources from counselors, therapists, and sex therapists to help you overcome obstacles and achieve your goals.

Remain Dedicated: Despite setbacks or obstacles, remain dedicated to the process of improving your marriage's intimacy and sexual satisfaction. Recall that improvement takes time, and that every step you take will bring you and your partner closer to a more meaningful and profound connection.

Continue to Learn: Look for opportunities to learn and develop in your sexual relationship on a regular basis. Maintain your curiosity, try out novel concepts and methods, and be willing to change as a couple.

Give Your Relationship Top Priority: Put your relationship and the health of your partnership first above all else. Give your relationship with your partner the care and attention it deserves in order to lay a solid foundation for a lifetime of intimacy and love.

Applying the knowledge from "Sex in Your Marriage" and making a commitment to the development and enhancement of your sexual bond will help you and your partner have a more lively, rewarding, and profoundly satisfying relationship.

Bonus

Description of the ratings;

1= Very extremely unsatisfied

2= Extremely unsatisfied

3= Unsatisfied

4= Not cool

5= Do not care what I feel

6= Not sure what I feel

7= Just cool

8= Satisfied

9= Extremely satisfied

10= Very extremely satisfied

Note: Use an erasable pencil to enable you to revisit the worksheet.

Sexual Satisfaction Inventory

Instructions:

▫Offer sincere and distinct answers to every question.

▫Take your time to reflect on your feelings and experiences in your sexual relationship.

▫After finishing the inventory, discuss your answers with your partner to pinpoint your areas of strength and potential improvement.

▫Make use of this as a springboard for candid conversations about your desires and level of sexual satisfaction.

Questions:

▫How happy are you with the frequency of sex in your relationship, on a scale of 1 to 10?

_____ (1-10)

▫To what extent are you happy with the way you and your partner communicate about sex?

_____ (1-10)

▫Score your happiness with the diversity and originality of your sex encounters.

_____ (1-10)

▫To what extent are you happy with the emotional intimacy and connection that occur during sex?

_____ (1-10)

▫Score your happiness with the way your sexual relationship strikes a balance between giving and receiving pleasure.

_____ (1-10)

▫To what extent are you happy with the amount of experimentation and willingness to try new things in your sexual encounters?

_____ (1-10)

▫How comfortable and trusting is it for you to talk to your partner about your sexual desires and boundaries?

_____ (1-10)

▫To what extent are you happy with the general sense of fulfillment and satisfaction you get from your sexual relationship?

_____ (1-10)

Reflection:

▫After finishing the inventory, pause to consider your answers.

▫Think about the aspects of your sexual relationship that are working well and the ones that might use some work.

▫Consider what concrete steps or adjustments you can take to improve your sexual gratification and strengthen your relationship with your partner.

Discussion:
▫Set aside some time to discuss your answers with your partner.

▫Tell your partner the truth about your feelings and thoughts, and encourage them to do the same.

▫Use this as an opportunity to discuss your sexual desires, preferences, and concerns, and to identify areas where you can work together to improve your sexual relationship.

Action Plan:
▫Make an action plan to address any areas of concern and strengthen your sexual relationship's strong points based on your discussion.

▫Determine clear objectives and benchmarks, and pledge to assist one another in achieving increased intimacy and sexual satisfaction.

With the help of this Sexual Satisfaction Inventory worksheet, you can evaluate and enhance their sexual relationship and promote increased closeness, fulfillment, and connection.

Fantasy Exploration Worksheet

Introduction:

A normal and healthy part of human sexuality is fantasizing. You can increase intimacy, strengthen your bond, and liven up your sexual relationship by discussing and exploring your fantasies with your partner. This worksheet is intended to assist you in exploring and talking about your shared sexual fantasies.

Instructions:

Take turns completing each section of the worksheet on your own, then get together to share and talk about your answers with a partner. Be open-minded, curious, and considerate of each other's fantasies and boundaries as you approach this exercise.

Fantasy Identification:

▫Jot down three arousing or intriguing sexual fantasies or scenarios. These may be long-standing fantasies or ones that have just come to you.

Fantasy 1:

Fantasy 2:

Fantasy 3:

,,..

▫Please rate your comfort level in sharing each of your fantasies with your partner on a scale of 1 to 10.

Fantasy 1: _____ (1-10)

Fantasy 2: _____ (1-10)

Fantasy 3: _____ (1-10)

„..

Fantasy Discussion:

▫Start by discussing the fantasy you feel most comfortable discussing with your partner when you share your fantasies. Give a thorough description of the fantasy, mentioning the characters, the setting, and the activities.

Partner A's Fantasy:

Partner B's Reaction/Feedback:

„..

▫Talk about the parallels and discrepancies among your fantasies. Are there any recurring themes or components that both of you find intriguing? Do you both want to explore any particular fantasies together?

Discussion:

„..

▫Examine the bounds and possibilities within every fantasy. Does one partner find any aspects of the fantasy uncomfortable? Exist any boundaries that must be agreed upon or respected?

Boundaries/Limits:

„..

Fantasy Integration:

▫Select a fantasy that the two of you can explore together with ease. Talk about integrating aspects of this fantasy into your romantic partnership. Would you like to try any particular scenarios or activities? How can you make both partners' experiences safe and enjoyable?

Fantasy to Explore:

Integration Plan:

„...

▫Think back to the time you spent discussing and sharing your fantasies with your partner about sex. What was the experience of disclosing your desires? Did it strengthen your bond or give you fresh ideas for a sexual partnership?

Reflection:

„...

In summary:

Adding more intimacy and connection to your sexual relationship can be achieved by completing this fantasy exploration worksheet. Recall to approach this exercise with candor, transparency, and consideration for one another's boundaries and fantasies. You can strengthen your relationship, stoke passion, and open up new possibilities for satisfying and exploring your sexual fantasies by talking about and exploring them together.

Sensate Focus Exercises

Introduction:

One of the most effective ways to improve intimacy and pleasure in your sexual relationship is through sensual focus exercises. Through these exercises, one can concentrate on touch sensations without feeling compelled to perform sexually or experience an orgasm. You can improve communication, establish trust, and strengthen your physical bond by engaging in sensate focus exercises together. Using a series of sensate focus exercises, this worksheet will lead you through discovering and appreciating touch in a fresh and meaningful way.

Instructions:

Work through each exercise with a partner, switching between being the touch provider and receiver. Establish a dedicated time slot and make sure the space is distraction-free and cozy. Be open to connecting on a deeper level and approach each exercise with an open mind.

Exercise One: Non-Sexual Touch Exploration

■ Maintaining relaxed posture and eye contact, both of you should sit or lie down facing each other.

■ Alternately use your fingertips, palms, or hands to gently touch various parts of your partner's body. Without anticipating being sexually aroused, concentrate on investigating the tactile sensations.

■ As the one being touched, be aware of how each touch feels and let your partner know how you're feeling. When describing the feel and quality of the touch, use precise language.

■ After a few minutes, take turns letting your companion examine your body in the same manner. Encourage candid feedback and open dialogue throughout the exercise.

Exercise Two: Progressive Sensate Focus

■ Start with both of you lying down in a comfortable position, either fully or partially clothed.

■ As the giver, begin by touching your partner lightly and gradually increase the pressure and intensity as you go.

■ Pay attention to feeling around your partner's body in both erogenous and non-sexual areas.

■ As you examine your partner's body, encourage them to share their preferences and feelings with you. To direct your touch, pay attention to both verbal and nonverbal cues.

■ Change places and let your partner be the one providing the touches after a predetermined amount of time. As the recipient, practice being receptive and actively listening.

Exercise Three: Mutual Sensate Focus Massage

■ Create a cozy environment with massage oil or lotion, calming music, and soft lighting.

■ Alternately massage each other sensually, emphasizing pleasure and relaxation.

■ To warm up the muscles, begin with long, sweeping strokes and then progressively add more concentrated pressure and techniques.

■ Throughout the massage, encourage your partner to share their preferences and feelings. Utilize both spoken and nonverbal cues to direct your touch and modify your method as necessary.

■ Spend some time together thinking back on the massage experience after each partner has had a turn giving and receiving one. Talk about your experiences, your favorite parts, and any realizations or learnings you had from the exercise.

You and your partner may have a profoundly transformative experience by completing these sensate focus exercises, which will improve intimacy and strengthen your physical bond. Always remember to approach each exercise with curiosity, openness, and a desire to jointly explore novel sensations. Frequent practice of sensate focus can help you develop a better understanding of each other's bodies, boost pleasure and satisfaction, and fortify your relationship.

Desire Mapping Worksheet

Introduction:

A fulfilling and satisfying intimate relationship is largely dependent on your ability to understand your sexual preferences and desires. Through the process of "desire mapping," you can discover and map out your desires, fantasies, and boundaries. Using a series of questions and prompts, this worksheet will assist you in mapping out your sexual desires and sharing them with your partner. Together, you can strengthen your bond, increase intimacy, and build a more satisfying sexual relationship by completing this exercise.

Instructions:

After finishing each worksheet section on your own, get together with a partner to share and discuss your answers. Be open-minded, truthful, and respectful of each other's boundaries and desires as you approach this exercise. Take advantage of this to strengthen your bond as a couple and to gain a deeper understanding of each other's sexual needs and preferences.

Section One: Turn-Ons

▫Name three things that reliably make you feel aroused or lustful.

a)

b)

c)

▫Explain the particular traits or attributes that you find most appealing in your partner.

a)

b)

c)

Section Two: Turn-Offs

▫Name three things that make you feel less attracted to or sexually inclined.

a)

b)

c)

▫Determine any actions, situations, or behaviors that cause you to feel uneasy or nervous when having sex.

a)

b)

c)

Section Three: Fantasies and Desires

▫Give an example of a sexual scenario or fantasy that you find especially alluring or thrilling.

▫Consider any fantasies or desires you've been afraid to discuss with your partner. What has prevented you from expressing these desires?

Section Four: Boundaries and Limits

▫Determine any limits or boundaries you have regarding your engagement in or enjoyment of sexual activities. These could be boundaries that are emotional or physical, or they could be particular actions or behaviors that make you uncomfortable.

▫Talk about any traumatic or past experiences that might have affected your current limits or boundaries. In what ways can your partner help you uphold and respect these boundaries?

Completing this worksheet on desire mapping is a critical first step in improving communication and intimacy in your sexual relationship. Take advantage of this chance to discuss your fantasies, boundaries, and desires with your partner. Pay close attention to their answers. You can strengthen your bond, experience more pleasure and fulfillment, and develop a more satisfying sexual relationship by encouraging open and honest communication.

Intimacy Building Activities Worksheet

Introduction:

Creating emotional intimacy is a prerequisite for building a solid and fulfilling relationship. Intimate ties, which foster mutual trust, understanding, and intimacy between partners, are the cornerstone of a happy and healthy partnership. This worksheet provides a series of activities designed to increase closeness and fortify your bond with your partner. Together, by completing these activities that will improve communication and fortify your bond, you can create intimacy and fulfillment in your relationship.

Instructions:

Work through each exercise with a partner, switching roles as the participant and the initiator. Allocate a specific period for these pursuits and establish a cozy, carefree atmosphere that fosters candid dialogue and emotional bonding. With an open mind, curiosity, and a desire to strengthen your relationship with your partner, approach each activity.

Activity One: Sharing Gratitudes

■ Each of you should say three things about your relationship for which you are thankful. These could be little things, deeds of kindness, or traits you value in your spouse.

Partner A's Gratitudes:

1.

2.

3.

Partner B's Gratitudes:

1.

2.

3.

■ After exchanging thanks, talk about how being grateful improves communication and fortifies your bond. Consider the advantages of valuing and recognizing one another's contributions.

Activity Two: Mindfulness Practice

■ Select a comfortable sitting or lying position, then turn to look at each other while keeping your eyes open.

■ Together, take a few deep breaths in and out of your body, paying attention to how the breath feels coming and going.

■ Set aside some time to engage in mindful breathing exercises, allowing yourself to be fully present and be aware of one another's presence.

■ After the mindfulness exercise, discuss your thoughts and feelings with your spouse. Discuss how practicing mindfulness together improves your relationship and makes you feel more intimate.

Activity Three: Non-Sexual Touch

■ Make time for your partner to touch you in a non-sexual way. This can involve giving each other massages, holding hands, or cuddling.

■ Pay attention to your partner's physical touch and the physical connection between you.

■ Take turns describing your feelings and how the touch makes you feel. When expressing your feelings and sensations, use detailed language.

■ Discuss the experience collectively after the touch session. Talk about the ways that non-sexual touch builds emotional ties and increases intimacy.

Conclusion:

By completing these intimacy-building exercises, you and your partner can develop a closer, more meaningful relationship. Make better use of this worksheet to help you develop intimacy, communication, and a deeper bond in your relationship. You can build a more loving, understanding, and trusting partnership by regularly participating in these activities together.